Handbook of Mental Health Nursing

Edited by
Stephen Tee, Joanne Brown and Diane Carpenter

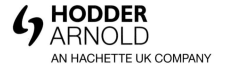

HODDER
ARNOLD
AN HACHETTE UK COMPANY

First published in Great Britain in 2012 by
Hodder Arnold, an imprint of Hodder Education, a division of Hachette UK
338 Euston Road, London NW1 3BH

http://www.hodderarnold.com

British Library Cataloguing in Publication Data
A catalogue record for this book is available from the British Library

Library of Congress Cataloging-in-Publication Data
A catalog record for this book is available from the Library of Congress

ISBN-13   978-1-4441-2129-2
1 2 3 4 5 6 7 8 9 10

Commissioning Editor: Naomi Wilkinson
Project Editor: Mischa Barrett
Production Controller: Francesca Wardell
Cover Design: Lynda King

Cover image © Masaaki Kazama

Typeset by Datapage India Pvt Ltd
Printed and bound in Spain

What do you think about this book? Or any other Hodder Arnold title?
Please visit our website: www.hodderarnold.com

We dedicate this book to Tina, Alison and Lucy, who found time to contribute to this book their experiences of mental health care so that others can learn

Contents

Contributors

Karen Ainsbury M Inst GA UKCP
Group Analytic Psychotherapist
and
Supervisor and Organisational Consultant
Bournemouth, UK
Member of the Institute for Group Analysis

Marion Aslan
Executive Director, Elemental;
Chair, Elemental Wellbeing
Coventry, UK

Joanne Brown BA MA PhD
Senior Lecturer in Mental Health, Faculty of Health Sciences
University of Southampton, UK
Member of the British Association for Counselling and Psychotherapy

Diane Carpenter RMN DipN(Lond) DipNEd(Lond) BA(Hons) MSc PhD RCNT RNT
Lecturer in Mental Health, Faculty of Health Sciences
University of Southampton, UK

John Carthy RMN Fe tec MA
Consultant Forensic Nurse
London, UK

Tina Coldham
PG Cert in Strategic Social Care Leadership
Service user consultant
Winchester, UK

Lucy Davies HND RMN
Service user consultant
Portsmouth, UK

Helen Eunson RMN MA PGCE
Practice Development Nurse and Training Lead
Southern Health NHS Foundation Trust
Hampshire, UK

Alison Faulkner Bsc(Hons) Msc
Service user consultant
London, UK

KWM (Bill) Fulford DPHIL FRCP FRCPSYCH
Fellow of St Cross College

and

Member of the Philosophy Faculty and Honorary Consultant Psychiatrist
University of Oxford

and

Emeritus Professor of Philosophy and Mental Health
University of Warwick

and

Former Adviser for Values-Based Practice to the National Mental Health Development Unit
Department of Health
London, UK

Gwyn Grout RMN MSC PHD
Independent Consultant Nurse
Guildford, UK

Judith A Lathlean DPHIL (OXON) MA BSC (ECON)
Professor of Health Research
Faculty of Health Sciences
University of Southampton, UK

Chris McLean BA DIP N RN (ADULT) PCAP
Lecturer in Nursing
Faculty of Health Sciences
University of Southampton, UK

Jane Pritchard RMN BSC(HONS)
Consultant Nurse
Northamptonshire, UK

Julie Repper RGN RMN BA(HONS) MPHIL PHD
Associate Professor and Reader in Mental Health and Social Care
School of Nursing and Midwifery
University of Nottingham

and

Service User and Carer Engagement Fellow
Collaboration for Leadership in Applied Health Research and Care (CLAHRC)
Nottinghamshire, Derbyshire and Lincolnshire

and

Recovery Lead
Nottinghamshire Health Care Trust
Nottingham, UK

Mike Smith RMN Bsc(Nurs) MA PhD
Director, Crazydiamond
Liverpool, UK

Stephen Tee RMN DPSN BA MA PGCEA DclinP
Head of Centre for Innovation and Leadership in Health Sciences
Faculty of Health Sciences
University of Southampton, UK

Wendy Turton RMN RNMH Bsc(Hons) Bsc(Hons) (Thorn Accredited) Msc BABCP
Clinical Lead
Psychosocial Interventions for Psychosis Service
(PSIPS)
East Area
Southern Health NHS Foundation Trust

and

CBT Lecturer and Clinical Supervisor
CBT Centre
School of Psychology
University of Southampton, UK

Acknowledgements

We would like to thank the following: colleagues and students at the university of Southampton Faculty of Health Sciences; Tina Coldham, Alison Faulkner and Lucy Davies for their invaluable time, input and support; Lotika Singha for excellent copy-editing; and Mischa Barrett, Project Editor, and Naomi Wilkinson, Commissioning Editor, at Hodder Education for their patience and for keeping us on track.

Part 1

The Philosophy and Practice of Mental Health Care

Stephen Tee, Joanne Brown, Diane Carpenter, Tina Coldham, Lucy Davies and **Alison Faulkner**

Introduction

Introduction to relational mental health nursing

This chapter aims to help you, the reader, appreciate the complex nature of mental health nursing. To this end we have included a number of personal accounts from three of the authors of this chapter who have experience of using mental health services. These accounts describe what it is like to receive mental health care so that you will begin to understand what it means to work with people experiencing mental health problems.

These accounts are not always flattering to mental health nursing, but do tell us something important about what people want and need from mental health services and, most importantly, what they do not need. These accounts have been chosen as, although they do not always paint mental health services in a positive light, we feel it is important to learn from examples where poor practice happens so that we can develop appropriate values, skills and attitudes that will give you the confidence to challenge poor practice and improve services.

Experiences of emotional distress and mental health nursing

Case Study 1.1

Alison's account (see also Faulkner 2005, 2010)

I have been admitted to acute mental health wards on a number of occasions: perhaps about seven or eight times between 1998 and about 2005, never for

continued ➤

longer than six weeks and usually less. During that time I had some good experiences and a great many not so good experiences.

On the first occasion, in January 1998, the ward manager shook my hand when I was admitted and said something like 'I'm sorry that things are not so good for you right now'. He was a big and gentle man, who I also observed defusing some difficult situations. On that same ward, however, I observed or experienced many incidents of what I can only call abuse.

There is, perhaps, a fine line between poor or inadequate treatment and abusive treatment. Once you are admitted, hospital routines prevail and daytime television may be the main activity until the next ward round, which may well be cancelled without notice and you are lucky if anyone tells you in advance. It is commonplace not to be given information, or to be given inaccurate information. On one admission it was five days before I found out who my key nurse was, and the information sheet I was given about admission was mis-spelt and appeared to be out of date and inaccurate. It stated that the use of mobile phones was forbidden on the ward and yet both staff and patients were using them indiscriminately.

On one occasion, I was sitting in the non-smoking TV room, as was my key nurse. He turned to me and said 'So, have you ever slept with a man, Alison?' I could not believe that he was prepared to open such a conversation with me in a public area, and was rendered speechless.

I watched one patient being shouted at for accidentally leaving the ward to go to the canteen early because he thought it was lunch-time. He was threatened and grabbed by nurses. It was easy from my position to see that he had simply left the ward following someone else – perhaps an unlabelled member of staff – thinking that they were on the way to the canteen.

Another event that was significant to me was the time when I watched a nurse taunting two male patients with the accusation 'You poofs, you poofs!' They were both pacing up and down the ward and had started to hold hands as they paced. The nurse turned to me for approval or support. I got up and left, unable to challenge him.

After a few years, the wards were segregated by gender and I was admitted to a women-only ward. Ironically, the treatment was worse in some ways. Some of the nurses were used to the ward being a rehabilitation ward and consequently seemed bent on getting us to get up early and make our beds. I felt aggrieved about this as I did not feel that I had come into hospital in order to learn how to make my bed.

On one of these occasions, there was a nurse on duty who was forever shouting orders at us ('Make your bed!' 'Medication time!' 'Get up – you can't stay in bed all day!'). On one occasion she shouted at a man for taking his cup of tea from the dining room towards the smoking room: 'You finish your drink in here!' He shouted back at her, and the spat showed every sign of escalating, at which point I intervened. Why shouldn't he take his tea through to the smoking room? 'Because you all leave cups all over the ward, it's a mess.' (This was in a ward where we couldn't get hot drinks at other than the specified times.) She said to me 'I'm not shouting at you, am I?' and turned her attention towards me. I was not very brave. I wanted to say that the rule was ridiculous, or that if she had talked differently to him, treated him with some respect, the whole situation would have been different. But I said nothing more.

On one occasion, I was standing behind an older woman in the queue for medication. She was someone I had only ever seen eating her meals with some enthusiasm or quietly watching television. When offered her medication, she put it in her mouth but refused the cup of water to swallow it down with. The nurse told her to take the water, and she refused again. This time the nurse began to shout at her: 'Swallow your pills; have you swallowed it? You've got it in your mouth still haven't you? Open your mouth, open your mouth!' With this, she pointed her finger threateningly and close to the woman's mouth. This continued for some minutes. The nurse said that she would record the woman's 'non-compliance' in her notes.

Another time I was lying on my bed and overheard a nurse threatening a patient (who was crying) with transfer to the secure ward. Bravely, I got up and asked her what she meant: did crying mean that we would be transferred to a secure ward? No, she said – but that patient gets angry and throws things when she gets upset. I said nothing more. Again I was too scared to take this further but the outrage built up inside me. The only thing to do each time this began to happen was to get out as soon as possible.

On one occasion, after a doctor had told me 'You just can't cope with your life, Alison', I had to go and lie on my bed and repeat mantra-like to myself what I believed other people, my friends, thought about me, in order to repel his words.

It is some years now since I had these experiences, and I can only hope that things are better in most acute wards. One of the things I learnt during that time was that hospital could be a sanctuary for me but only for a very short time – perhaps a week or two at the most. After that the indignities of it would overwhelm me. It was a bad period. The hospital I was often admitted to also seemed to be poorly maintained – sometimes there would be no soap or toilet paper, no lock on the shower door or a broken toilet seat. As mentioned earlier, you could not get a hot drink outside of set times.

The difficulty with these experiences is not necessarily that they are bad in themselves, but that they perpetuate your low self-esteem and worthlessness. This

continued ➢

is not an environment in which recovery can be supported or promoted. It is hard to describe and important not to underestimate the extreme lack of confidence and fear of retribution that can accompany your role as a mental patient.

On the plus side, I had an excellent GP [general practitioner] in those early days, a man who was prepared to give me time almost every week if I needed it and who treated me with absolute respect at all times. Until recently I had a very good psychiatrist – again someone who treated me with respect. Far better than my experiences in hospital were my experiences with a crisis and home treatment team. Again, there was an element of respect and individualized care that made the whole thing more palatable.

Respect is more important than many of us realize. Recently I read a brief article by Professor Richard Warner (2011) (*The Stigma Inside Us*, www.scottishrecovery. net/Latest-News/the-stigma-inside-us.html) in which he lists a number of studies which demonstrate that insight alone is not enough to aid recovery. People with a strong internalized stigma are less likely to have positive outcomes, whether or not they demonstrate insight and acceptance of their condition. Warner finishes with the following sentence: 'They need to be treated with the respect that will allow them to retain a sense of dignity and to be provided with opportunities for advancement that will show them that they are masters of their own destiny.'

This certainly rings true for me. Periodic mental distress of most kinds can plunge you into a pit of despair, worthlessness and humiliation, often without the help of other people. What you need around you are people who believe in your ability to crawl out of that hole again and know how to communicate that to you.

Respect goes to the heart of mental health services and treatments, in my view. If we can respect each other, we can begin to treat each other with a common humanity. Institutions can so easily lose this fundamental principle that I can only believe they are inherently inhuman.

Case Study 1.2

Lucy's account

I have experienced mental health problems for the past 10 years; in that time I have been hospitalized a number of times, sometimes detained, others informally, in private and NHS [National Health Service] hospitals. In the community I have been cared for by a CMHT [community mental health team] at times with a care co-ordinator or via outpatients. I have experienced psychological therapies services and a crisis resolution/ home treatment team. I have had ECT [electroconvulsive therapy] and been prescribed medication from every relevant drug group in the BNF [British National Formulary]. I continue to take medication and have a diagnosis of schizo-affective disorder.

I think it is important to start by saying that any given intervention at any given time may be positive or negative depending on my state of mind at the time. That is to say, what I need or find helpful today, I may not tomorrow. I have also found whilst thinking about what to write that elements of care, particularly those which I have found helpful, are quite hard to pin down and demonstrate. The experience is quite subjective, and care is truly a craft encompassing knowledge, experience, sensitivity and intuition, and different for each individual, both patient and staff. The things that haven't gone so well I have found are much easier to define and explain.

Continuity seems to me to be the thread that joins together all of the positive experiences I have had, from being admitted to hospital to long-term, well-established relationships with staff in the community.

Being an inpatient in a psychiatric unit can be scary; being admitted to a familiar place with faces you recognize goes some way to mitigate that. Over a number of admissions the scary place had become something of a sanctuary. I think this became the case because I felt listened to and understood. I felt that staff made a positive effort to spend time with me, which was not rushed or pressured. When I was scared the staff continually offered reassurance and when necessary would just 'be' with me; it was not so frightening with someone else there, I felt safer. I had the time to build trusting relationships–the qualifications or grades of staff weren't very important. I found the most helpful staff were those who were honest, empathic, gentle and encouraging, prepared to spend time with me, not necessarily 'doing' any spectacular intervention but just being.

On a more practical note, being in hospital involves a lot of waiting, ward rounds, medication, meals, etc. It's really helpful if things happen when they are supposed to, or if they are not going to happen that you are informed. I have often found it difficult to remember information that I have been given; it may need to be repeated or better still give me pen and paper! It was helpful for me to have quiet places to go as well as communal areas. Optional organized activities ranging from distraction to intensive therapeutic input were useful. The issue of medication and its place within psychiatry is a complex and controversial one. I have a great deal of ambivalence regarding its use. However, I can say that for me the opportunity to disappear into the oblivion of medication at times has been a welcome relief from the experience of acute distress, although sedation is not a long-term solution. Having opportunities to go outside and take a little exercise has also proven to be therapeutic, ensuring Section 17 leave is viable and within the ward's capacity is essential. And perhaps most importantly constant access to tea! I appreciate many of these points may be beyond your control but remembering what it is to be human and humane is probably a good start.

continued ➤

Less helpful are noisy and chaotic places. I was once on a ward that had a large sign in the lounge saying 'Do not spit on the floor'. I knew that this was going to be a different experience! I was allocated a named nurse on arrival; she went on two weeks' leave the next day. I was instructed not to leave the ward; as the dining room was on a different floor I didn't eat for three days until I summoned up the courage to ask a staff member for some food. He was only identifiable as a member of staff by his alarm and ridiculously large bunch of keys. Access to doctors was limited to a weekly ward round which appeared to involve every staff member in the hospital and was not conducive to any sort of therapeutic engagement.

There were a lot of agency staff and communication seemed poor across all of the staff, it felt that at any moment complete chaos might break out. The staff seemed under pressure, constantly 'fire fighting' and appeared to have no time. There was nowhere quiet, the TV being audible at all times, regardless of the fact that no one ever seemed to be watching it. In the chaos one rule was rigidly maintained: no hot drinks between midnight and 6 a.m. A low-flying book flung by a woman who had wanted a cuppa for a couple of hours did hit me but it was 5 a.m. She then activated the fire alarm and was later arrested for wasting the emergency services' time, for the sake of a cup of tea! Mysteriously, day or night there were always fewer cups than people. Fortunately, I was on my way quite quickly, being transferred to another hospital. The most caring act that I recall was a taxi being arranged.

In conclusion I would suggest that a number of small, considered and quite ordinary gestures accumulate to give an impression of care and being cared for. It is always worth remembering that you could one day be in my shoes.

Case Study 1.3

Tina's account

I sometimes think that my use of mental health services has been somewhat unremarkable. There are plenty of upsetting and harrowing accounts of which I have heard and find deplorable. I am a bog standard depressive, with some anxiety thrown in at bad times to pep things up a bit. I don't attract that much attention from self-harming or acting on suicidal thoughts. I don't behave oddly in public. I have learned to contain my distress and manage this at home. I am stable on the medication if I don't get stressed out by work and life, which happens frequently. I can afford to buy good-quality counselling privately, which is never available at the time I need it, in the style I want it, on the NHS. I have learned to manage my distress, which is still very real for me, all the time. This doesn't mean that I won't turn to services if in need – I will. I hope I can manage that interaction rather than it being imposed upon me.

I have two psychiatric careers. One I fell into from falling apart and the other paid worker role I've grown from the first. This is in order to put something back into the debate about mental health from a user perspective. How we respond as a society, and in turn how services respond to distress. Some of my passion comes from challenging the deplorable.

I realize now that I was first unwell but undiagnosed when in my mid-teens. My father had died of cancer, my brother's eyesight was failing, mother was struggling to cope with all this, home was not a happy place, and school was even worse. In my late teens I was put on beta-blockers by my GP, and then good old Valium [diazepam] for the anxiety and panic attacks I was experiencing. It wasn't until I was 25 that I became severely depressed and entered psychiatric services. More Valium and shedloads of anti-depressants. I was lucky though as I was treated at a psychiatric day hospital. I had made a new happier home for myself so didn't need inpatient treatment. The multi-disciplinary input at the day hospital served me well to give space to my distress, begin to understand my diagnosis, and tackle it with expression and self-management tools. After a year of treatment I made tentative steps back to work. After this, I remained an outpatient, requiring various levels of input until I graduated back to primary care after 17 years of secondary psychiatric service use.

Having said I keep a low profile, I can pinpoint moments of intervention that are both good and bad and stand out for me. There was the time that I went to see the duty psychiatrist, who, after forgetting I was coming, not being able to find my notes, and then after a scant read of them when found, fiddled with his pager whilst telling me that ECT was the best thing for me. This was the first time I had been offered this treatment, and he disagreed with me over the well-known side effects. Not for the first time I looked frantically for an escape route. Then there was the time a retired social worker who was a work colleague sat on me to stop me leaving my house at the dead of night in my dressing gown in a state of acute distress. Perhaps not the recommended control and restraint, but it did the job without hurting me. The on-call GP administered a large dose of Valium as all the beds at the local inpatient hospital were full. A narrow escape here. Then there was the time in a therapy group when I giggled at a trust exercise we were doing. I was very nervous and it came out like that. The senior nurse chastised me like a child for my apparent laughter. I disengaged mentally from the exercise after that, my fragile self-esteem crushed.

On a more positive note, I also remember the time when a nurse held my hand in A&E [accident and emergency] after I had taken an overdose of said Valium. We talked a little while. It turned out that she was on a higher dose of Prozac

continued ➤

[fluoxetine] than me! She connected with me with honesty and humility, whilst still being professional and getting the job done. The simple kindness of making me a cup of tea, I needed fluids anyway, compared favourably with the brusqueness of the doctor treating me, who was evidently fed up with timewasters not deserving his expert attention. I may have been 'shot away', but even in crisis, acutely depressed or under the influence of whatever, one can experience a true caring connection with another human being, and be aware when one is being rebuffed.

I remember the look of relief on the face of the nurse who had come to my home to see if I was still alive after failing to get me on the phone. The line was down it transpired, and she was worried about me after my recent overdose attempt. Had I done it again? This time I could repay the effort by making this nurse a cup of tea, whilst she managed her own anxiety. Perhaps it was the thought of not having to fill out a serious untoward incident report, but she looked genuinely glad to see me and reassured us both that I was alright.

There was the time at the day hospital that I had a major crisis and was curled up in the corner of a room lost in my own grief. I had missed lunch, and two nurses kept popping in to see me, they gave me space but let me know they were there for me. Did I want something or someone? I later moved to the small garden and took a couple of paracetamol for my raging headache. A nurse's head appeared around the door to enquire about the exact dosage. Keeping me safe, showing they cared.

I do feel that the basis of good interventions is when people really show they care for you. Of course you have to keep a professional detachment; otherwise you would go mad too. This is the art of 'nursing' that you carefully hone during your career. But genuinely attempting to connect to someone, and to give a little bit of yourself whilst accepting and not rejecting the person in front of you, is the most powerful medication you can administer. It is not rocket science. Why is it that we talk about the 'Dignity Challenge'? Can we not treat others with dignity and respect when they are at their lowest or when in greatest need? I know I am seemingly not always the most grateful and receptive at the time, but the effort of the caring nurse getting through stays with you always. It can save lives.

So now, unless I'm being paid for my user insight, you won't find me in mental health services. I am considered too well for them nowadays, and this suits me fine. However, on the balance of probabilities, I will need to seek help from services again during my life. I hope to find honesty and pragmatism alongside a healthy dose of caring connection. I need someone to walk beside me and see me through the maze of my distress, holding my hand, literally or otherwise. Someone who values me for who I am, and can help me to put myself back together again. A challenge for me and those who work with me. A challenge worth working on.

Challenging practice

The above powerful and at times distressing accounts teach us a number of lessons about how it must feel to be admitted to a mental health unit and the vital role that communication, professional behaviour, safety, respect, decision-making and organizational culture have in the delivery of mental health nursing care.

It is poignant to think that more than 50 years ago Foucault (1961), reflecting on Western society, argued that institutions such as mental hospitals were expressions of medical (and nursing) power exerted over people in marginalized groups, such as mental health service users, by the dominant group, in this case nurses and doctors. Whilst Foucault was writing in the 1960s about the Victorian asylum system, a system which has largely been replaced by modern community-based services, it is rather disheartening to see that service users continue to experience similar attitudes and treatment in the twenty-first century. In addition, this book is written at a time of great resurgence in secure provision and increases in the prison population of people with mental health problems. The 'institutions', whilst no longer Victorian, remain present in a different form, and still feature prominently in the spectrum of provision for those people who choose, or are required by law, to use psychiatric services.

Although you personally may not recognize the experiences reflected in these accounts, the reality is that many in mental health nursing have embraced the prevailing discourse and accepted the dominant psychiatric position. Thus their 'clinical effectiveness' becomes narrowly focused on the relief of symptoms, the administration of medication and maintaining control rather than taking account of wider aspects of the individual's life (Seed house 2000).

This problem is compounded by the fact that, once someone is diagnosed and classified as vulnerable, the 'system' can sometimes maintain its surveillance and control of the individual in perpetuity. Foucault (1961) explained this thus:

> *Unreason ... is judged ... in order to be recognised, judged, classified and made innocent forever. It is caught ... in a perpetual judgment, which never ceases to pursue it and to apply sanctions, to proclaim its transgressions, to require honourable amends, to exclude, finally those whose transgressions risk compromising the social order.*

(p. 255)

Barnes and Bowl (2001) echo this view, suggesting that the judgement made on service users is in sharp contrast to the perception of professionals as: 'healthy, competent and rational' (p. 128).

Seedhouse (2000), commenting at the start of this century on the prevailing culture of mental health nursing, suggested that practice contributes to this divide between the nurse and service user by highlighting and emphasizing erroneous behavioural responses and couching them in demeaning terms such as 'attention seeking', 'lacking insight' or 'a management problem' with little mention of the positive characteristics of the individual. This separation becomes even more apparent when mental health practitioners use mental health legislation to detain an individual against their wishes. At this point, Seedhouse (2000) argues, the nurse becomes: 'the police. No more, no less' (p. 137).

Nurses and the wider profession need to reflect on why, having undertaken professional training which purportedly acknowledges multiple models and discourses on mental health, and emphasizes a range of therapeutic approaches and promotes partnership working, their practice becomes demeaned to methods of surveillance and control which promulgate oppression and social exclusion. Linde (1993) suggests that it is the narrative which explains how personal and professional identity is constructed through the stories told and how these stories are shaped by cultural, institutional and national meta-narratives. Consequently the nurse, and student nurses on placement, working within a mental health system can become influenced by the dominant culture of psychiatry, the institutionalized system of the NHS and the policy directives from government and professional bodies which contribute to individual professional identity.

When professionals such as nurses encounter clinical situations, their decisional responses, according to Ledema (1994), become institutionalized. Over time nurses recognize a familiar situation and their response will be an uncritical acceptance of a particular worldview. The values and beliefs, which contribute to the shared meaning within such a culture, may be implicit or explicit and are, according to Brown (1998), deep manifestations of workplace culture. The problem, according to Kotter and Heskett (1992), is that changing culture at a deep level does not happen rapidly, or without challenge, as values are often hidden. Some have suggested that cultural change can take years (Williams *et al.* 1993).

Therefore if mental health nurses aspire to adopt an emancipatory stance in the process of clinical decision-making, as suggested in the new Nursing and Midwifery Council (NMC 2010) standards, then individual practitioners will need to critically examine their values, adopt a more sceptical position and challenge the dominant discourse; therefore challenging its validity, examining their workplace culture and contributing to a process of cultural change. This could include examination of the current uncritical acceptance of the rational, medical discourse to explain the nature of the person's experience which underpins many mental health nursing texts and curricula, which seem out of step with nurses' aspirations to work in partnership and value diversity.

A humanitarian profession

The service user accounts clearly illustrate the need for an individual and person-centred approach to care that is sensitive to changes in a person's life. Preserving an individual's autonomy is a central tenet of professional practice, to ensure that individuality, personal integrity and choice are maintained. They highlight the importance of extending basic humanity to an individual experiencing distress and preserving dignity when someone is at their most vulnerable.

Hildegard Peplau (1952), known as the mother of mental health nursing, described nursing as:

a significant, therapeutic, interpersonal process. It functions co-operatively with other human processes that make health possible for individuals in communities ... Nursing is an educative instrument, a maturing force, that aims to promote forward movement of personality in the direction of creative, constructive, productive, personal and community living.

(p. 16)

What Peplau is saying here is that the essential characteristic of nursing is the creation of a shared experience, established through the skills and techniques of observation, assessment, formulation, interpretation, decision-making, validation, planning and intervention. At the simplest level through listening to the client, the nurse will develop a general impression of the person's circumstances and will then seek to validate their interpretations through a checking process to determine accuracy. The service user accounts above highlight the importance of the four domains of practice identified by the NMC. Nurses must care, they must develop effective inter-personal and communication skills, they must be competent and they must be able to take appropriate evidence-based decisions and be able to lead and to work with others.

Our responsibilities as professional practitioners

The regulatory body which oversees nursing is the Nursing and Midwifery Council, established in 2002. The NMC's stated purpose (NMC 2002) is to 'safeguard the health and wellbeing of the public' (www.nmc-uk.org). Its core functions are to:

- Register nurses and midwives and ensure that they are properly qualified and competent to work in the UK
- Set the standards of education, training and conduct that nurses and midwives need to deliver high-quality health care consistently throughout their careers
- Ensure that nurses and midwives keep their skills and knowledge up to date and uphold the standards of their professional code of practice
- Establish fair processes to investigate allegations made against nurses and midwives who may not have followed the code of practice.

In order to meet these functions the NMC publishes a wide range of guidance for professionals, employers and the public explaining the standards nurses are expected to achieve. To carry out effective practice, the judgements exercised by the nurse need to be informed by an explicit set of contemporary professional values that unify practice around a common set of behaviours. These are not the same as the institutionalized values described earlier. It is also important for nurses to appreciate the philosophical underpinnings of their profession and be conversant with the values and performance expectations to which all nurses are expected to subscribe.

An interdisciplinary profession

Uniquely the body of 'evidence' for mental health nursing is derived from a wide range of disciplines across the life and social sciences. These sciences can include psychology, sociology and biology, and will combine to help the nurse fully understand the different dimensions of an individual's health care needs. Mental health nursing is rarely carried out in isolation, and nurses need to learn to work at the interface where disciplines come together to plan, implement and review treatment and care. A nurse's co-workers will typically include psychiatrists, psychologists, social workers, occupational therapists and general practitioners, but this list should also include family members, employers and other community groups. This is a point illustrated in UK policy, which emphasizes the notion that mental health is 'everyone's business'.

The cross-government mental health outcomes strategy for people of all ages *No Health Without Mental Health* (Department of Health (DH) 2011) highlights the need for everyone, including individuals, families, employers, educators and communities, to contribute to good mental health. It outlines six shared objectives:

1. More people will have good mental health
2. More people with mental health problems will recover
3. More people with mental health problems will have good physical health
4. More people will have positive experience of care and support
5. Fewer people will suffer avoidable harm
6. Fewer people will experience stigma and discrimination.

Within the DH (2011) strategy some important statistics are highlighted:

- At least one in four people will experience a mental health problem at some point in their life; and one in six adults has a mental health problem at any one time.
- One in 10 children aged between 5 and 16 years has a mental health problem, and many continue to have mental health problems into adulthood.
- Half of those with lifetime mental health problems first experience symptoms by the age of 14, and three-quarters before their mid-twenties.
- Self-harming in young people is not uncommon (10–13 per cent of 15–16-year-olds have self-harmed).

- Almost half of all adults will experience at least one episode of depression during their lifetime.
- One in 10 new mothers experiences postnatal depression.
- About one in 100 people has a severe mental health problem.
- Some 60 per cent of adults living in hostels have a personality disorder.
- Some 90 per cent of all prisoners are estimated to have a diagnosable mental health problem (including personality disorder) and/or a substance misuse problem.

These statistics illustrate the diversity of need and a requirement for highly skilled practitioners who can work with people of all ages. In this chapter we have attempted to identify the current context and challenges of nursing. By drawing on service users' experience we have emphasized the importance of the relational components of care. These themes will be further explored and developed in subsequent chapters.

How this book is organized

This book is organized in two parts. Part 1 focuses on you as an individual practitioner and encourages you to reflect deeply on who you are and on what kinds of philosophies, psychologies and values inform your practice. It asks you to think about how you behave in groups and about what recovery from mental health problems means to you. It conjoins theory and practice and encourages you to be reflective and curious about the different forces at work in your own life and practice. Part 2 looks at the broader system of mental health practice and at the socio-historical and political forces that have shaped the field of mental health nursing.

Throughout this book we will try to engage you in dialogue and speak to you directly. Theoretical positions are outlined, but it is not our aim to 'lecture' you, but to talk to you and to try to present theory with an illustrative example or a prompt for reflection. In this sense, we hope that the style of this book is Socratic and not didactic. These chapters have been written by educators and clinicians who have drawn on their practice and classroom experiences in order to draw you into a virtual conversation about who you are as a practitioner and what underpins your practice.

The chapters have been read by Alison, Tina and Lucy and they have looked at the extent to which these chapters stayed near to experience, even when explicating theory, or deviated from it. They helped us to think about whether what we felt it was important to 'talk' to you about as future practitioners was, in fact, important to what is needed to improve practice and change it where necessary. Of course, we have to be mindful of critiques of tokenistic service user involvement (see Chapter 9) and only they and you can judge whether we have been mindful enough. By asking Alison, Lucy and Tina to read these chapters and write about their own experiences, we have not intended to imply that we remain untouched by emotional distress and/or bad practice. We have not, however, chosen to write from our own personal experience in these chapters and perhaps this is an unequal practice that is worthy of challenge. We have written from our position as educators and clinicians, while hopefully staying close to the idea that, as Lucy said, one day it could be (or has already been) me or you who is vulnerable and in need of compassionate and skilled care.

In this book our aim has been to encourage you to adopt a psycho-social approach to mental health nursing and to look at individual, familial and inter-personal dynamics as well as looking at groups, institutions, discourses and histories of mental health nursing. The thematic continuity uniting these chapters is in their emphasis on de-stigmatizing feelings of pain and despair and bringing them back into their rightful place as part of the human condition. Philosophers and psychologists through the ages have looked at anxiety, frailty and the suffering we can inflict on each other as an intrinsic part of what it means to be human. Thinking about our very humanity as being a source of suffering, as well as a source of intense joy, might not be an easy mirror to hold up to ourselves, but by doing so we might be less inclined to stigmatize people for whom life has become a source of suffering. Moreover, there are many people who would not delete their history of emotional distress, despite the strength that is needed to survive it.

Part 1

Chapter 2 outlines generic reflective practice exercises and introduces a skills-based approach to psychological theories which can help you to develop a therapeutic use of self. Most of them involve looking at your own distress, destructiveness, pleasures and life-affirming qualities because you will need to tune in to who you are, and what you feel, in order to understand and reach out to the other. This chapter is more than twice as long as the other chapters in this book because it discusses a subject that is crucial to mental health studies and practice: the therapeutic use of self. Chapter 3 similarly asks you to be reflective, but it also asks you to not just focus on your personal values but also how these may relate to your professional values, and the values of those you work with. You might see links between Chapters 2 and 3 and identify ways in which your values are affected by the values of those who you grew up with, or you might see ways in which your own history attracted you to the professional values you associate with mental health nursing.

Chapter 4 is also concerned with reflective practice, but you are now asked to pan out to the larger group and think about what groups mean to us and what habitual position we adopt (the charismatic leader, the quiet observer, the joker and so on). You will probably work with groups at some point and it is important to be able to understand what anxieties and hopes people bring to groups and how you can best facilitate them.

Chapter 5 brings you the voice of people in emotional distress and asks you to think outside of the context of services and therapeutic interventions in order to aid recovery (to family, friends, communities and so on). The point is made that we can only understand what recovery means if we listen to people who have had catastrophic experiences and begun to feel less crushed by them. The continuing stigma around mental health problems is highlighted and this may well affect you too. How might you feel if you start to feel depressed, for example whom would you tell? This relates back to Chapter 2 and the importance of 'wounded healers' and others telling of their own emotional pain and difficulties as a means to normalize psychic distress. Chapter 5 demonstrates that recovery does not involve looking for a cure (for the human condition?), but for a way to make life bearable when hope is wilting. The way in which the concept of recovery has been appropriated by services and academics is discussed in this chapter and in Chapter 8 in Part 2.

Part 2

The chapters in this part of the book do not ask you to reflect as deeply on your personal qualities, values and expectations, and instead focus more on practice and the politics of practice. Chapter 6 introduces you to evidence-based practice and its importance and relevance is explained. It is acknowledged that empiricism is not the only form of knowledge (as we see in Part 1), but evidence-based practice is essential to your future career. You are given a step-by-step guide to working through how to gather evidence for your practice and for implementing changes. Implementing change is not easy, but, if you have developed your own personal skills (perhaps by completing some of the exercises in Part 1), you will be in a much better position to anticipate resistance and understand how to navigate it and what it might make you feel.

Chapter 7 has detailed guidance on how to increase your confidence and competence in decision-making via working through four case studies. Here you will be asked to use both intuition and logic in order to make informed decisions about care. You are given a reflective guide for practice which will enable you to provide a rationale for the decisions that you take and you will be able to use the skills learned in the previous chapters in order to provide full and meaningful answers to the question of why you have worked in a particular way.

In a similar way, Chapter 8 will introduce you to the concepts of management and leadership in mental health nursing and will help you to differentiate between them in order to enhance your future leadership and management roles. You may want to refer back to Chapter 4 on groups and think about your predisposition to leadership or back to Chapter 2 to think about histories of leadership or management in your family. Your inter-personal skills will be crucial if you want to develop the clinical expertise in your area and empower staff; and this chapter takes you through what it means to be led or to lead. You might want to reflect on whether you will make a good leader or manager and on why management is often denigrated, while visionary leadership is applauded. Both, as this chapter outlines, are central to good quality care and to implementing progressive changes.

In Chapter 9 we ask what it means to promote health and social inclusion in wider society. That is, how do we implement change at the level of services *and* at the level of society? Answering this question involves looking back at the history of nursing and this makes for uncomfortable reading at times. You will be asked to think about aspects of care that have changed and those that have not. Moreover, you will be asked to think about the language of mental illness and our response to those who do not conform to our normative assumptions about mental stability or health. In this chapter you will be asked to think about what you expect from those you work with (a modicum of stability or signs of vital growth?) and about what you are doing to nurture a person's capacity to thrive.

Here we find that the role of the mental health nurse is inherently politicized and you are invited to think about how you will develop that aspect of your role. For example, to what extent does the history of mental health nursing and some examples of practice now trouble your own values base? This chapter warns about the tokenistic and confused attempts at social inclusion in some cases, and we are encouraged to work towards equal service user integration into services and society, rather than a polite invitation to institutional bodies where the power base remains unchanged. You are asked to think about what you expect from the people you work with, and what recovery, thriving or social inclusion mean to you.

Chapter 10 ends the book by asking you to finally consider what mental health nursing was in the past, what it is now and where you would like to see it in the future. You will be challenged to think about what defines your profession now and what defines you as a practitioner. For example, are there different types of mental health nurse – the psychological therapist, the political advocate, the nurse as service user, the researcher nurse, the nurse scientist, the spiritual nurse? We can think of any number of permutations and this book asks you to think about the context in which nursing has evolved and about what informs your practice. This means taking up an interested and questioning position in relation to your profession and practice area and rather than adopting an unquestioning identification with dominant cultures or discourses of health, illness, therapy and evidence and so on. It is not easy to question a dominant status quo and when doing so you might encounter cultures of resistance (Main 2001). Change threatens us all and it is not easy to be the bearer of change, but neither is it easy to work in static, unchanging and defensive cultures.

References

Barnes M, Bowl R (2001) *Taking over the Asylum: Empowerment and Mental Health*. New York, NY: Palgrave.

Brown A (1998) *Organisational Culture*, 2nd edn. London: Pitman Department of Health.

DH (2011) *No Health Without Mental Health: A Cross-Governmental Mental Health Outcomes Strategy for People of All Ages*. London: Department of Health.

Faulkner A (2005) Institutional conflict: the state of play in adult acute psychiatric wards. *Journal of Adult Protection* **7**(4), 6–12.

Faulkner A (2010) Measuring the marigolds, in Basset T, Stickley T (eds) *Voices of Experience: Narratives of Mental Health Survivors*. London: Wiley-Blackwell.

Foucault M (1961) *Madness and Civilisation*. London: Routledge.

Kotter JP, Heskett JL (1992) *Corporate Culture and Performance*. New York, NY: Free Press.

Ledema R (1994) *The Language of Administration: A Detailed Description of the Literacy Demand of Administration and Bureaucracy*. Sydney: NSW Department of Education.

Linde C (1993) *Life Stories and the Creation of Coherence*. New York, NY: Oxford University Press.

Main T (2001) Knowledge, learning and freedom from thought, in Day L, Pringle P (eds) *Reflective Enquiry into Therapeutic Institutions*. London: Karnac.

NMC (2002) *Code of Professional Conduct*. London: Nursing and Midwifery Council.

NMC (2010) *The Code: Standards of Conduct, Performance and Ethics for Nurses and Midwives*. London: Nursing and Midwifery Council. Online: www.nmc-uk.org/Nurses-and-midwives/The-code/ (accessed November 2011).

Peplau H (1952) *Interpersonal Relations in Nursing*. New York, NY: GP Putman's Sons.

Seedhouse D (2000) *Practical Nursing Philosophy*. Chichester: John Wiley & Sons.

Warner R (2011) *The Stigma Inside Us*. Glasgow: Scottish Recovery Network. Online: www.scottishrecovery.net/Latest-News/the-stigma-inside-us.html (accessed November 2011).

Williams A, Dobson P, Walters M (1993) *Changing Culture, New Organisational Approaches*, 2nd edn. London: Institute of Personnel Management.

Joanne Brown

The therapeutic use of self

Learning outcomes

- Be able to reflect on the concept of a therapeutic use of self
- Understand the challenges of providing evidence of efficacy and outcome measures for the therapeutic use of self
- Be able to look at the therapeutic use of self from the humanistic, psychodynamic or cognitive behavioural perspectives
- Reflect on your role in developing a therapeutic use of self

Introduction

The aim of this chapter is to highlight the way in which reflective practice is at the heart of a therapeutic use of self. This chapter is divided into four sections. Section 1 provides a discussion of the generic concept of reflective practice and its importance in mental health practice. It will introduce you to reflective practice exercises and to their limitations. Section 2 provides a discussion of some basic tenets in humanistic psychology and offers exercises and examples of reflective and therapeutic practice in action. Section 3 provides an overview of major concepts in psychodynamic psychology and includes exercises which will enable you to increase your understanding of what a therapeutic use of self refers to within this approach. Section 4 offers you an understanding of some of the basic reflective tools that are commonly used in cognitive behavioural therapy (CBT). Given the ubiquity of CBT, it is assumed that you might be more familiar with this philosophy and technique and only a broad overview is given.

Throughout all four sections, the aim is to enable you to develop your understanding of reflective practice and to see how it is central to developing a therapeutic use of self. You will be able to deepen your understanding of a reflective and therapeutic use of self and hopefully be able to begin to: (1) think about which therapeutic and philosophical approaches are best suited to your practice and (2) identify situations when you might move between these different approaches. The aim of this chapter is to therefore enable you to develop your theoretical and practical understanding of the different ways in which a reflective and/or therapeutic use of self can be conceptualized and put into action.

Section 1: the art and evidence of reflective practice

Mental health nurses must have and value an awareness of their own mental health and well-being. They must also engage in reflection and supervision to explore the emotional impact on self of working in mental health: how personal values, beliefs and emotions impact on practice, and how their own practice aligns with mental health legislation, policy and values based practice frameworks.

(Professional values 8.1, Nursing and Midwifery Council (NMC) 2010 Competency Framework)

The UK NMC (2010) competencies for mental health make repeated references to the therapeutic use of self as being central to a nurse's ability to promote mental health and wellbeing. This chapter aims to discuss what the therapeutic use of self entails, and it will begin with the *New Shorter Oxford English Dictionary*'s (Brown 1993) definition of the word 'therapeutic':

The branch of medicine that deals with the treatment and cure of disease and ill-health; the art of healing. A curative agent; a healing influence. Also loosely, health giving, relaxing, stress-reducing.

(p. 3274)

What the therapeutic use of self therefore suggests is that we need to use who we are as a healing influence in our relationships with clients. It implies that it is our capacity to make a relationship with another person and also end it sensitively that has a curative effect.

Researchers at the Centre for Outcomes, Research and Effectiveness (CORE) at University College London (UCL) have produced a map of competencies (based on empirical evidence of efficacy) for cognitive behavioural, psychodynamic and humanistic clinical practice. However, they also note that 'successfully engaging the client and building a positive therapeutic alliance is associated with better outcomes across all therapies' (Lemma *et al.* 2011, p. 15).

Although you might not train to be a therapist or counsellor, the therapeutic use of self (as we have seen from the NMC competencies) is central to mental health nursing. Peplau's (1952) classic psychodynamically informed text *Interpersonal Relations in Nursing* casts nursing as, in one important respect, 'relationship therapy' (Reynolds

2003). Of course, Peplau recognized that the conditions that support processes of self-repair and self-renewal are psycho-biological (physiological as well as inter-personal), but her book focuses on the inter-personal skills that nurses need to deploy in physical and emotional care. Interestingly and perhaps controversially Peplau (1952) stated that:

> The basic task of the school of nursing ought not to be 'concern for the patient', which is the task of a nursing service; the task of the school of nursing is the gradual development of each nurse as a person who wants to nurse patients in a helpful way.
>
> (p. xi)

That is, your mental health training ought to offer you time for relational, experiential learning as well as academic, evidence-based learning. As Johns (2004) explains:

> If you consider that 'who I am' is the major therapeutic tool I use in my practice, then clearly I need to know myself well in order to use myself in the best therapeutic way. Reflection is about coming to 'know who I am', so I can refine and sharpen this tool for therapeutic work.
>
> (p. 37)

The psychoanalyst Bion (1970) referred to therapists being able to develop a kind of binocular vision which would enable them to easily move between external and internal landscapes. Deploying this skill as a mental health nurse would mean that you need to be able to pan out to the external world of research, policy and politics and back in to your own values, feelings, history and life path.

Evidence-based practice

There are, according to Johns (2004), cognitive and aesthetic approaches to reflective practice. A therapeutic use of self might be seen to belong to the aesthetic approach (an art rather than a science), but this does not mean that it cannot be used to provide evidence-based outcomes (see Chapter 6 for a discussion of evidence-based practice). Indeed there is a plethora of research looking at the therapeutic alliance and treatment outcomes in different client populations. For example, Shirk *et al.* (2008) have looked at the predictive relations between therapeutic alliance and outcomes in CBT for adolescent depression, Karver *et al.* (2008) have studied alliance-building behaviours and treatment outcomes in youth psychotherapy, and the link between the therapeutic alliance and outcome has also been studied in the context of couple and family counselling (Mahaffey and Lewis 2008) and bipolar disorder (Berk *et al.* 2008). Street *et al.* (2009) have more generally considered whether and how communication is linked to health outcomes, and Keen and Lakeman (2003) point to various positive patient outcomes that are correlated with an effective therapeutic alliance. More broadly, the importance of empathic communication to better health outcomes is studied in contexts other than mental health (see Hopkinson *et al.* (2011) for a systematic review of psychological interventions for families where one member has advanced cancer).

Papastavrou *et al.* (2011), however, argue that 'there is still scarcity of literature and systematic evidence about how caring interventions can enhance patient outcomes and help them to deal with the stress of illness more effectively' (p. 1). They provide a systematic review of nurses' and patients' perceptions of caring behaviours in order to test the hypothesis that nurses and patients perceive the concept of caring differently. They argue that we need more research on which client group, for example, might value the instrumental, technical (know-how skills) more than expressive, affective and psychological skills, and vice versa. That is, nurses' and patients' expectations about therapeutic care might vary according to the setting they are in (from psychiatric care to critical care and whether the nurse is a man or a woman, etc.). They explain that in one study in their systematic review (von Esen and Sjoden 1993):

> somatic and psychiatric patients differed in their perception of caring behaviours as the task-oriented aspect of caring was rated as more important from patients hospitalised in medical and surgical settings … patients with mental health problems considered the cognitive aspect of caring as the most important aspect of care.

The authors acknowledge the limitations of their review (it is of quantitative research only with limiting inclusion criteria), but it is cited to alert you to ways in which perceptions of and the need for therapeutic care might vary, and to the ways in which a relational phenomenon which is difficult to isolate is subjected to evidence-based enquiry.

However, differentiating technical (biophysical) and relational (psycho-social) aspects of care is problematic (see the von Esen study above) and it is not only people with mental health problems who need to be treated in a way which is psychologically and empathically skilled. The public outrage (see Abraham 2011) at the way in which older people are treated has been fired by incredulity at how fellow feeling is lost in any setting (be it mental health or physical health) where a professional neglects or abuses a person who is suffering and vulnerable. Indeed Freshwater and Stickley (2009) argue that therapeutic care is in danger of being marginalized in a climate that disproportionately promotes evidence-based care over values-based care:

> Where once the therapeutic relationship was the primary focus of mental health practice (Altschul 1997; Barker 1999; Peplau 1952) more recently it has become marginalised in favour of tangible interventions.
>
> (p. 30)

Johns (2004) similarly explains that a functional perspective on nursing (which defines nursing practice in terms of what people do) prevails, rather than a philosophical perspective (which defines practice in terms of the practitioner's beliefs and values). He argues that nurses can feel under pressure to support the medical task (with an emphasis on observable behaviour and outcomes), and thereby neglect the emotional, psychological, spiritual and social aspects of nursing. It is for this reason that researchers at CORE acknowledge that the method that they have adopted for gathering evidence of efficacy in order to produce a map of competencies is not without its critics. They cite two significant objections, for example, made by humanistic practitioners:

- The evidence base places an inappropriate focus on techniques of therapy, to the neglect of 'relationship' factors.

- The standard of evidence that CORE has adopted is almost invariably the randomized controlled trial. Roth *et al.* (2011) explain that 'there is a view that such trials need to be supplanted by qualitative approaches, or trials which are more process-oriented, and that both these methods can validate the efficacy of an approach as conclusively as the RCT' (p. 10).

Reflective practice

Johns (2004) charts the many existing reflective models (Carper 1978; Casement 1985; Gibbs 1988; Mezirow 1981; Schon 1987), including his own model for structured reflection, but what he is keen to emphasize is that, although reflective practice might be a 'reflection-on-experience' (Schon 1987), the ultimate aim of reflective practice is to develop a kind of practical wisdom that is based on becoming mindful or self-aware. The *New Shorter Oxford English Dictionary* (Brown 1993) provides us with the following definition of reflection:

> The action of turning back or fixing the thoughts on some subject; meditation, serious consideration. Recollection, remembrance. The process or faculty by which the mind has knowledge of itself and its workings.
>
> (p. 2521)

Reflective practice is central to psychological therapy, mindfulness and emotional literacy, and also to more politicized, socio-historical thinking in the form of critical theory and scholarship. I have written elsewhere (Brown 2006) about a 'psycho-social imagination' as a particular form of reflective practice which combines sociological and psychological sensibilities. Separating the psychological from the sociological self is artificial, of course, since the very discourse of a therapeutic use of self is saturated by its own socio-cultural and historical specificity (see Furedi (2003) for a critique of therapy culture). This chapter, however, will focus more on how we might develop our self-reflective and relational skills, rather than deconstruct why this discourse of the therapeutic prevails. Nevertheless, it is important to deploy a 'sociological imagination' and question what hierarchies of knowledge exist and how these affect what you might feel able or unable to do in training and practice. A sociological imagination will help you to look at what kinds of practice, therapies and nursing care are valued, and why.

Freshwater and Stickley (2004), for example, are critical of the dominance of evidence-based practice in nursing research and training, and they write about authors like themselves who want to rehabilitate the emotions and the importance of fostering emotional literacy and intelligence in nurse training. Freshwater (2004) quotes Orbach's

(1999) definition of emotional literacy as 'the capacity to register our emotional responses to the situations we are in and to acknowledge those responses to ourselves so that we recognize the ways in which they influence our thoughts and our actions' (Freshwater 2004, p. 14). In order to do this we need to be self-reflective, mindful and interested in our relations with others. Emotional intelligence is a similar concept for which Bar-On (2000) was the first to develop a test, but it was Goleman (1995) who popularized the concept. However, Freshwater notes that, despite becoming an international bestseller, it still has not had a significant impact in nurse training.

The new UK NMC (2010) competencies do make repeated references to the therapeutic use of self and to self-reflection as being central to the future of leadership and management in nursing:

> 4.1 Mental health nurses must actively promote and participate in clinical supervision and reflection, within a values based framework, to explore how their values, beliefs and emotions affect leadership, management and practice.

However, Johns (2004) is careful to warn us about the dangers of turning something that is essentially about a way of being into a programmatic way of doing:

> It is easy to get locked into the technology of reflection, 'how to do it', simply because we live in a technological world that demands explanatory models.
>
> (p. 42)

He argues that aesthetic expression and a more narrative approach to fostering reflective practice balance the more cognitive approaches to reflection that might currently exist in nurse education. Smythe (2004), for example, argues that 'reflective practice in nursing is too readily measured by the yardstick of positivism' (p. 326). Freshwater and Stickley (2004) also warn against reducing communication skills training to the science of the technician. That is, what they refer to as transformatory learning cannot be prescribed via orderly steps and they point out that self-enquiry is not always comfortable and it may stir up strong feelings.

Smith (1999), who has written about nursing as a form of emotional labour, argues that 'the modern jargon about self … abounds with optical and cerebral metaphors like "perspective", "viewpoint", "construct", etc.' (p. 154). Smith, however, also argues that emotions are 'full-on, urgent, fulsome, ghastly, glorious and gutsy'. She quotes Milton's *Paradise Lost* ('The mind is its own place, and in itself can make Heav'n of Hell, a Hell from Heav'n'; Smith 1999, p. 154) in order to remind us of the power of feeling. Prescriptive reflective practice models do not necessarily help us to connect with, express or evoke the emotional power of our relationship to our self and others. Hence Johns (2004) describes painting his feelings about the death of a patient, rather than answering pre-determined questions in a reflective practice model, and he cites many ways of facilitating reflective practice, including listening to each other's stories (so-called campfire teaching). Indeed Barker (1999) maintains that 'telling stories is the stock-in-trade of psychiatric and mental health nursing' (p. 3); and, interestingly, the word conversation, Schultz (1986) explains, is derived from the same Latin root as 'conversion'. The possibility of a 'conversion, of a turning around' is, Schultz says, 'inherent in any true conversation' (see Fromm 1986, p. 89). The 'art of conversation' (see Freshwater and Stickley 2006; Zeldin 1995) like any other craft requires practice.

This chapter will encourage you to engage in reflective practices which can facilitate emotional literacy and develop your therapeutic use of self. The exercises can be done alone or in groups. An experienced group facilitator can carefully observe how this work is being done and help to facilitate a safe environment with clear ground rules. You also need to keep yourself safe and be observant of how to protect the safety of those you work with. We will begin with two generic reflective exercises and then move on to look at how we might use some of the insights from the three major schools of psychology (psychodynamic, humanistic and cognitive behavioural) for more specific types of reflective practice.

Exercises in self-reflection and speaking and listening

Reflective Exercise 2.1

A window into the soul

Consider the Johari window in Table 2.1. Take a piece of paper and draw a square with four quadrants like in the table, but vary their size according to how open, hidden, blind or unknown you feel now compared with, for example, five years ago.

You can use these 'windows' to look at who you are and to talk about the differences between who you are now and who you were five years ago. You do not have to go into detail and, if you prefer, you could just do this on your own. Remember that you will be asking clients to talk to you about who they are and some practice at doing this yourself will hopefully increase your understanding of what it is like for them. You cannot, of course, draw this window to exactly mirror your levels of self-awareness, but you can vary the quadrant sizes in order to suggest how open, blind, hidden or unknown you feel yourself to be. A close friend, partner, therapist might construe it differently and this is also interesting to consider. Look at 'Julie's' use of the Johari window in Tables 2.2 and 2.3 and then draw your own.

After drawing your own window consider the following questions:

- Are you more open and self-aware now than you were, for example, five years ago (quadrant 1)?
- Do you find that people point things out to you about what you're like that you might initially find hard to see (quadrant 2)?
- Are you very hidden or private (quadrant 3)?
- Do you think that there are vast areas of your mind and feelings that are unknown by you and others (quadrant 4)?
- Does your answer to any of the questions above depend on who you're with or the setting you are in? Give examples.

- Do you feel comfortable with self-disclosure and do you know how to manage appropriate boundaries around what you disclose?
- How did you feel about doing this?

Table 2.1 The Johari window

1. Open/free area	2. Blind area
3. Hidden	4. Unknown area

1. What is known by the person him/herself and is also known by others.
2. What is unknown by the person about him/herself but which others know.
3. What the person knows about him/herself that others do not know.
4. What is unknown by the person him/herself and is also unknown by others.

(Source: Luft and Ingham 1955.)

Table 2.2 Julie: five years ago

	Known to self	Unknown to self
Known to others	*Open*: Julie (22 years old) is very depressed and does not see many people or go out. She does not understand why she feels so bad. On the outside, Julie appears cheerful and friendly, but inwardly she does not respect herself and feels lost. She would like to have children, but fears she never will be able to, because of relationship problems	*Blind*: Julie's friends tell her that she is being possessive and jealous with her partner and with them. Julie can't see it and thinks that they are excluding her. When she's drunk she starts arguing with them and pushes them away
Unknown to others	*Hidden*: Julie tries to hide from people, because she feels as though they will just look down on her. She avoids going out unless she's had a drink and she feels very alone with a hidden, denigrated self	*Unknown*: Julie feels as though there is a vast area of her that is unknown and that neither she nor other people can see

Table 2.3 Julie: now

	Known to self	Unknown to self
Known to others	*Open*: Julie now feels like she can be more open about who she is and she feels much more self-aware than she was five years ago when she was very depressed, she did not like herself and she did not see other people or go out. Five years ago, she wasn't aware of how self-defeating and deeply rooted her negative thoughts and behaviour were, but now she has more understanding of how her own past, thoughts and feelings have affected her life. She is now more hopeful about having children	*Blind*: Julie's blind spots are fewer now. She is open to trusted friends telling her if she isn't seeing something that they can (she's choosing the wrong partner or drinking to excess or pushing people away)
Unknown to others	*Hidden*: Julie is less hidden from people now, because she hates herself less, but she doesn't 'wear her heart on her sleeve' and she is circumspect about whom she talks to	*Unknown*: Julie still feels like there are large parts of herself out of her conscious awareness and she wants to look into this more by continuing to write in her diary and take time to be mindful and reflective

O'Shaughnessy (1994) explains that the self has an old wish for omnipotence, and this can make it difficult to look sympathetically at our blind spots and mistakes and learn from looking at them. Children, for example, can feel humiliated and belittled if they get something wrong, because it might trigger a despair about the self and feelings of being worthless, stupid and unlovable. As adults, we are not immune from these feelings of shame or humiliation if we feel exposed or lacking, and reflective practice can, therefore, be challenging. Hence Cooper (2003) asks:

> Is it possible to engage in true learning from experience without some element of critical self-reflection? ... We all have a capacity for self-criticism, but this can take on a more or less helpful form, depending upon whether it is a spur to self-examination and reorientation of our thinking about ourselves or self-immolation and despair about our own worthlessness.

(p. 56)

It is, therefore, important to establish ground rules if reflective practice exercises are done in a workshop setting, but these rules won't necessarily inoculate us against the power of our feelings.

Reflective Exercise 2.2

Listening, being listened to and observing

Let yourself associate freely to any of the prompts below. Do this in a reflexive journal or with trusted peers. If you do this with peers, in groups of three, select one person to be the observer, one to be the speaker and one to be the facilitator. The speaker has 10 minutes to use one of the prompts to freely associate to. The facilitator's role involves helping the speaker to talk for as long as they can about their chosen topic. The observer notes the verbal and non-verbal aspects of this interaction. Each person takes it in turns to be a speaker, observer and facilitator and at the end of this exercise you can give each other feedback on your verbal and non-verbal inter-personal skills. Obviously, if this is done in a journal, you cannot elicit this feedback, but the prompts might still increase your self-awareness (see quadrant 1 in the Johari window).

Yesterday I felt …

When I was a patient/client …

A peak experience for me was when …

I once worked with someone who …

My parents told me …

I'd really like to change the way that I …

I tend to approach people with …

My journey into this profession began …

This exercise gives you the chance to speak and be listened to and it gives you the opportunity to see how it feels to be a facilitator and to be observed.

You can reflect on when you hit points of resistance in yourself and stopped talking and think about whether this was because of some internal censorship or because your facilitator did or said something that made you feel self-conscious and inhibited. You might also reflect on what qualities in a facilitator help you to reflect and open up (the look in their eyes, the tone of their voice, whether they smile and when). As well as reflecting on your own facilitation style, you will be reflecting on your peer's facilitation style and be able to learn from observing them.

You will need to be careful when you give each other feedback on your reflective practice and communication skills, because you might touch on each other's blind spots or hidden self. I, for example, might like to think of myself as a gentle and empathic facilitator, but I may be told that I can convey something forbidding and inaccessible. If this observation is true and I am told in a way that is not accusatory, it will be a very important insight for me to have about myself. Below is a list of the kinds of things you might consider providing feedback on as an observer, speaker or facilitator.

Non-verbal communication

- See Egan's (2010) acronym SOLER (is the facilitator Sitting at a comfortable angle and distance, do they have an Open posture (legs and arms uncrossed), are they Leaning forward from time to time and looking genuinely interested and listening attentively, do they make effective Eye contact without staring, do they looked relatively Relaxed?)
- Humour – Is humour used? In what way is it used?
- Touch – Is touch used? In what way is it used?
- Mirroring – Do you notice the facilitator and observer mirroring each other's body language?
- Attentive listening – Does the facilitator nod, etc.?
- Silence – Is silence used? What effect does this silence have?
- Presence – Does the facilitator appear to be available or elsewhere?
- Tone, volume of voice – What kind of voice does the facilitator use and does the volume or tone change?
- Facial expression – What kind of facial expression does the facilitator have?
- Does the facilitator keep time and in what way?

Verbal communication

- Are open or closed questions used (some practitioners warn against an overuse of what, where, why, when questions)?
- Challenges – Does the facilitator challenge the speaker at all?
- Interruption – Does the facilitator interrupt the speaker?
- Interpretation – Does the facilitator try to interpret the speaker's feelings, behaviour, thoughts?
- Reflecting – Does the facilitator reflect on the feeling conveyed by the speaker?
- Does the facilitator use praise and in what way?
- Boundaries – Does the facilitator use self-disclosure and how?
- Ending – Does the facilitator keep a sense of time and prepare for the end of time?
- Facilitation style – Overall what is their facilitation style? (You could look up Heron's (1993) six-category intervention analysis and Jacob's (2000) guidelines on facilitation skills.)

The above exercises are designed in order to help you to become an observer of your own inner processes and in order to help you to reflect on how they affect your inter-personal relationships. Doing these simple exercises can help you to develop generic counselling or communication skills.

Section 2: philosophies of care – Humanistic psychology and person-centred care

Humanism, existentialism and phenomenology are the philosophical influences that one can identify in humanistic psychology or person-centred care and each will be briefly discussed here. The discourse of person-centred care pervades all branches of nursing and here we will unpack what this means.

Humanism

Humanism states that we are all equal by virtue of being human and that we carry our own individuality and all of humanity within us. As Fromm (1988) said 'nothing human is alien to me' (p. 77), and, in his book *Anti-Semite and Jew*, Sartre (1948) asks Shakespeare's question: 'If you prick me, do I not bleed?' Although the discourse of humanism has been deconstructed and challenged (see Davies 1997), we can see that the emphasis on egalitarian and collaborative relationships in person-centred care is informed by humanism. Mental health students who work with challenging behaviours might sometimes find this commitment to humanism challenging. How might you feel, for example, if someone screams at you and swears, or defecates or cuts themselves or tries to hit you? These are extreme examples, of course, and not all mental health clients present with this kind of behaviour, but you do need to anticipate having strong feelings stirred up in you and not necessarily liking what you see and feel.

Even if we do encounter behaviour that is alarming, humanists maintain that we should judge the 'sin and not the sinner' and they argue that human nature is good or neutral and that destructiveness, sadism, cruelty and malice are violent reactions against frustration of intrinsic needs, emotions and capacities (see Maslow 1962; Mearns and Thorn 2007). The Mearns and Thorn text will be used in this chapter in order to explore the creeds of humanism. It is also one of the texts used by CORE when it devised national competencies for humanistic therapy.

Mearns and Thorn explain that unconditional positive regard involves deeply valuing the humanity of your clients irrespective of particular client behaviours. The attitude, they say, manifests itself in the practitioner's consistent acceptance of and enduring warmth towards her or his client (Mearns and Thorn 2007). Can you think of a time when you have found it difficult to value the humanity of one of your clients and convey warmth (students in forensic settings sometimes find positive regard challenging, for example)? Do you think that this humanist creed is realistic or helpful to you in your practice? Can you hate what someone has done and still value their humanity?

Humanists also ask us to be congruent. Mearns and Thorn (2007) argue that congruence is the state of being when our outward responses to our clients consistently match the inner feelings and sensations which we might have in relation to the client. They provide the following example from humanistic counselling:

Do you really think you can help me?

(Long silence)

No ... no ... I can't see how I can help you [pause] it feels like you're so tied up by all that past experience, that it's difficult to know who you are, never mind knowing whether or not I can help you.

(p. 78)

Humanistic practitioners might be congruent and express confusion or irritation, but they must still practise unconditional positive regard. Congruence can diminish power imbalances in a relationship and facilitate trusting, egalitarian and companionable relationships in which open communication is valued. Being congruent and practising unconditional positive regard is consistent with the humanistic commitment to equal rights which is enshrined in nursing policy. The Department of Health's (2011) *No Health Without Mental Health* strategy document refers to the right to 'No decision about me without me'; and the service user movement in different contexts calls for collaborative person-centred care. However, it has to be recognized that, when we are overwhelmed by tormenting thoughts or feelings, we cannot always make decisions in our own best interests or accurately gauge what the other might be thinking or feeling.

Many professionals, artists, politicians, sportspeople (William Styron, Frank Bruno, Alistair Campbell and so on) have written or spoken about their own 'wounded souls' (see Rippere and Williams 1985) and this 'movement' also has a democratizing and normalizing effect, which can help to de-stigmatize emotional and psychological pain. Does your practice setting or role make it safe or appropriate to acknowledge that practitioners also experience mental health problems?

Humanistic psychologists do distinguish between self-disclosure and congruence. A congruent response, Mearns and Thorn (2007) explain, is a genuinely felt response to the client's experience at that time and is relevant to the immediate concern of the client. They provide the following example:

> *I remember when I lost a close loved one – I also felt that kind of 'desolation' which you have described, but you are saying something more … you are saying that as well as feeling desolation, you are feeling … a kind of … annihilation?.*

(p. 82)

Humanists ask us to practise with authenticity and they would argue that we and our clients have emotional antennae for incongruent behaviour which might involve, for example, a person looking bored with us, but offering help, being effusively warm, but seeming false, being charming to us, but it feeling manipulative. Does your practice setting allow you to work in a way which feels authentic? Are there times when incongruence is unavoidable?

Reflective Exercise 2.3

In congruence

Which of the following terms are descriptive of you as a person and of you as a mental health worker? Are there any words that you could add?

Creative	Intellectual	Spontaneous	Artistic
Loving	Strong	Warm	Forceful
Confident	Energetic	Quiet	Obedient
Aesthetic	Introverted	Sensuous	Understanding
Firm	Demanding	Aggressive	Shy
Humorous	Thoughtful	Polite	Genuine
Defensive	Fun-loving	Tender	Logical
Intense	Spiritual	Extroverted	Conforming
Judgemental	Sexual		

Which aspects of you 'as a person' do you not use in your mental health work? Is this justifiable or does it warrant review? (Taken from Mearns and Thorn 2007, p. 92.)

Phenomenology

Phenomenology is a philosophy about the nature of human experience and it is a method for immersing oneself in another person's experience of, for example, fear, abandonment or psychosis. Person-centred care emphasizes the importance of trying to understand the life world of another person, rather than 'viewing them through the lens of diagnosis and classification' (see Barker 2003, p. 4). Indeed Fromm (1994) argued that mental health practitioners should read novels in order to prepare for a training in mental health (rather than only prioritizing the *Diagnostic and Statistical Manual of Mental Disorders* (DSM)-IV, for example) and many mental health trainings do make good use of the arts and humanities in order to help students to empathize with, for example, the experiences of depression, anger, hope and resilience via film, poetry and literature.

Mearns and Thorn (2007) explain that empathy is a:

continuing process whereby the practitioner lays aside her own way of experiencing and perceiving reality, preferring to sense and respond to the experiences and perceptions of her client. This sensing may be intense and enduring, with the practitioner actually experiencing her client's thoughts and feelings as powerfully as if they had originated in him/herself.

(p. 39)

They give the following example:

He treats me like a baby–looking after me all the time, mollycoddling me all the time ... suffocating me! He fails to realise that since I've come to university I am not such a baby anymore ... I'm independent ... I'm strong.

(p. 43)

They then provide four levels of response beginning with the least empathic:

Level 0: Men are all the same.
Level 1: God, that must be hard.
Level 2: It's like he doesn't understand you ... how you're changing ... he still treats you like he used to, which may have been OK then, but not now ... and you're damned angry at that.
Level 3: I see your anger that he doesn't understand that you're changing ... that seems really really strong ... but I also wonder ... you look as though you're trembling ... is that trembling just your anger or is there something else going on in you as well?

Mearns and Thorn (2007) explain that level 3 'touches on the edge of awareness' (p. 44), for example, the client's fears about the loss of the relationship. Empathic responses are depth reflections which might pick up on sensations, felt sense, the flavour of something (tightness, darkness, falling, fog, etc.). It is this ability to attune to the other that is central to all therapeutic work, whichever modality you choose to work in. It is central to psychodynamic work, even though significant differences in technique and philosophy exist between psychodynamic and humanistic practice.

For the group analyst Craib (1994), for example, these depth reflections involve attending to 'the background noise to our encounters, a barely noticed feeling of comfort or discomfort' (p. 173). The seminal work of the developmental psychologist Stern (1985) involved studying the emotional attunement or 'mis-steps in the dance' between mothers and their infants. He argues that emotional attunement is one of the ways in which 'we can get inside of other people's subjective experience and let them know we have arrived there, without using words' (p. 138). Attunement does not lead to cognitive knowledge, but instead to a sense of communion. Wilkin (2003) similarly uses the notion of aligning with someone's 'tempo' to capture this sense of attuning to the other. He says that in order to develop a feeling of belonging with another you need to identify the other's melody and harmonize accordingly. Wilkin refers to the feelings, generated by the other, as the guiding light in achieving a sense of rapport and he states that:

> *Unless the nurse consults people and looks at life from their viewing gallery, they will fashion an object that is precious only to themselves.*

> *(p. 39)*

Wilkin (2003) asks you to consider how you create a climate of becoming. Is it the way you say things? Is it something you do or refrain from doing? Are you aware of such situations? What do you feel? Or do such situations become identifiable once they are over? According to Wilkin, the therapeutic use of self does not rely on a problem-or solution-focused approach, except insofar as it might involve thinking about why there might be an inability to achieve rapport. Wilkin (2003) quotes a letter from George, one of the 'inpatients' on a ward that he worked on, who had a psychotic breakdown, but had later recovered:

> *At one stage, I thought I had entered hell. It was the most frightening experience of my life. I felt tormented and terrified. I just could not understand why you had followed me there, but you had.*

> *(p. 41)*

Wilkin does not prioritize a particular therapeutic approach (CBT, cognitive analytical therapy, dialectical behavioural therapy, etc.), only his presence and making himself available to 'George' and his inner world. Although his work might be informed by a particular approach, he does not describe this, but instead focuses on his attempt to stay close to George's experience. And here we can see links to the phenomenological emphasis on understanding the world as the other experiences it. Indeed the new NMC (2010) competences also call for practitioners to:

> *value, respect and explore the uniqueness of people's lived experience of mental distress and recovery as an evidence base to inform practice.*

> *(Domain 1:2)*

Existentialism

Existentialism is a philosophy that emphasizes the importance of contemplating the fundamental facts of our existence (birth, the chance-like nature of life, death) as a way to live more decisively in the present. Sartre (1948), for example, argues that we are responsible for the meaning that we give to life (even, he contentiously said, behind barbed wire), but that we often use excuses in order to evade this responsibility. For example, we might stay in an unhappy relationship for years or live in the same area all of our lives and feel the passive victims of fate, rather than the active agents of our destiny. There are, of course, obstacles that might limit what we can do in life, but existentialists are keen to draw our attention to the ways in which we are afraid to choose how we want to live. Sartre said that the ultimate existentialist question has to be 'What have you made of your life?'

Existentialist psychotherapy (see Yalom 2001) makes a distinction between the everyday mode of existence and the ontological mode of existence. The everyday mode is when we are focused on the practical events of any day (breakfast, travelling, shopping, work, etc.) whereas the ontological mode is more philosophical (How long will I live for? Am I living life meaningfully? Who will my daughter grow up to be? How will I feel when a close relative dies?). Yalom argues that trainee therapists benefit from placements in a hospice setting in order to develop this ontological mode and to be able to enter into these kinds of conversation when clients need to.

Johns (2004) writes about his nursing work in a hospice setting and he argues for the importance of Watson's idea of trans-personal nursing (as a human-to-human encounter in which you might help people to find meaning in their suffering). He says that this moves nursing from the medical model to a world of existential suffering in which questions about what it means to be human are centrally important. Existentialists stress the importance of living in the present and warn against an unconscious fantasy that we are immortal. It is because we cannot contemplate our mortality that we do not live our lives decisively – a regret which people reflect on at the end of their lives:

> *Oh, I've had my moments, and if I had to do it over again, I'd have more of them. In fact, I'd try to have nothing else. Just moments, one after another, instead of living so many years ahead each day.*
>
> *(quoted by Kabat-Zinn 2005, p. 17)*

Reflective Exercise 2.4

What will you do with your life?

In *Thrive*, Aslan and Smith (2007) ask us to write a list of 10 things we want to do before we die. Here are some things trainees have told me:

- Have children
- Scuba dive
- Get married

- Get a doctorate
- Write a novel
- Be at peace
- Be a therapist
- Travel

I always then ask the question 'Are you going to do this, is it in your control?' and we talk about what obstacles we might foresee ('What if I'm infertile?', 'Would I adopt, foster?') and what steps we might take to navigate these obstacles.

Write your own list and think about whether you are moving towards doing the things that you want to do. You could review it in one year's time. This exercise can help you to think about whether you feel in control of your life (relatively speaking) and it can help you to have conversations with clients about whether they feel that their life is their own and how you might help them to 'seize the day'.

The above section gives you an example of the way in which humanistic psychology asks you to practise self-reflection. You could look at the CORE humanistic competencies (see www.ucl.ac.uk/CORE) and also read the case studies in Mearns and Thorn (2007) in order to think about whether there are aspects of humanistic psychology that fit who you want to be as a practitioner.

Section 3: philosophies of care – psychodynamic counselling

Freud's first model of the mind and therapeutic technique

> *Science and romanticism come together in psychoanalysis, but psychoanalysis to this day remains a scandal to the natural scientist as it also is to the Romantic.*
>
> (Symington 1986)

As already stated, we now have national competencies for psychodynamic therapy and you can look at them at UCL's website (www.ucl.ac.uk/CORE). Psychodynamic therapy or the talking cure is over 100 years old and what follows is a basic overview of some core concepts. It is an approach that has influenced contemporary therapies (for example, inter-personal therapy (IPT), mentalization, dialectical behaviour therapy and cognitive analytical therapy; it also has some affinities with mindfulness). Some authors would argue that its emphasis on that which is unconscious and relational make it less amenable to observable outcome-based research, but its evidence base for certain mental health problems (borderline personality disorder, for example) is established and growing (see Fonagy *et al.* 2007). Some of its philosophy and method also inform many of the therapies we see recommended in the National Institute for Health and Clinical Excellence (NICE) guidelines (IPT, family therapy, couples therapy, and so on).

Moreover, we are now said to live in a therapeutic, emotionalized culture (see Furedi 2003; Richards and Brown 2011) in which psychodynamic ideas are popularized (in chat shows, soaps and mainstream media). Psychodynamic therapy gives us language with which to understand the emotional and often unconscious communication that takes place between people and it argues that this emotional underworld influences many spheres of our life. Some of its basic tenets will now be explored.

The psychoanalytical view of the personality holds some similarities to the view of personality in the Johari window. That is, psychoanalysis states that there are three levels of mind – the conscious, pre-conscious and unconscious levels. The conscious is like quadrant 1 (an area of ourselves we are aware of). The pre-conscious is that which we are dimly aware of (things that are on the tip of the tongue, but are still slightly out of reach). The unconscious is like quadrants 2 and 4 (things the individual is unaware of about themselves, their behaviour and motivations). Our internal worlds are likened to a theatre (McDougall 1991) with its varied cast of characters and stories from over the years. This unknown area of the mind and its contents affect how we feel and behave, even though we may not always remember a dream or know why we feel envious, afraid, excited, irritated and so on. Freud said that 'in mental life, nothing which was once formed can perish' (1930, p. 256) even if, as Klein said, it only exists as a 'memory in feeling' (1957, p. 180). Hence these ancient memories in feeling can be the source of a *déjà vu* experience (triggered by a particular sight, smell or sound). The aim of psychoanalysis is to enlarge quadrant 1 or to bring more light into the room so that we can see and understand more of ourselves.

But there are resistances to self-knowledge and we may keep repressing feelings, thoughts and memories. *Resistance* and *repression* are key psychoanalytical concepts. Freud tried to bypass his patients' resistance and repression by *free association* – encouraging people to say whatever came into their mind (uncensored) and also by analysing their *dreams*. Dreams, he said, are the royal road to the unconscious. They are like messengers from our internal world and a form of self-dialogue that we can become attuned to. Freud initially believed that, if his patients could remember what they had repressed, their symptoms and mental suffering would cease and his early therapeutic method was therefore a cathartic (one patient said it was like chimney sweeping) talking cure.

Reflective Exercise 2.5

Rorschach Test and the Thematic Apperception Test (TAT)

You can download the Rorschach and TAT images from the internet. Choose a couple to look at, and in pairs take it in turns to free associate (say or write whatever comes into your mind).

- What does the inkblot remind you of?

Tell a short story using the TAT image as a prompt. Now reflect on what this might say about you and your current or past preoccupations.

- Does it reveal anything significant?
- Could you free associate?
- Did you censor yourself?

Freud's second model of mind and therapeutic technique

There are three structures in the mind according to this second theory:

1. The id is the amoral, instinctual, appetitive part of us and is full of aggressive drives and sexual urges and compulsions. It is irrational and driven by the avoidance of pain and anxiety and maximization of pleasure. It is an asocial aspect to us that needs to be held in check and contained, because it is narcissistic and egocentric.

2. The ego is the part of us that develops as we mature and tries to control our anti-social urges and be mindful of societal norms. Some have likened this part of us to an umpire or mediator.

3. The super-ego is our conscience and morality and is largely developed via early parental socialization. It is the part of us that can be judgemental and punishing (if we do something wrong) and is not always a benign part of the personality.

In dialectical behaviour therapy (see Baer 2006), the model of the reasonable, emotional and wise mind is also used, and here we can see similarities to the psychoanalytical view of the mind. It is the wise mind that is able to be in touch with reason and emotion simultaneously. It is both head and heart as Baer says. In psychoanalytical terms, this is referred to as the ability to think through feeling and it is a form of emotional intelligence or literacy which is central to psychodynamic work. Cooper (2007) says that in practice this means that you have a 'capacity to both absorb but also stay separate from the strong feelings that may be engendered (in service user, carers, family, professionals)' (p. 588) in your work. He adds that 'emotions are "intelligence" (i.e. information) not "disturbance" that tell you about the state of the whole system'. Hence, the psychodynamic approach helps us to be more in touch with our feelings and more aware of our thoughts, without becoming destabilized by them and acting them out (for example, by cutting, taking drugs, dissociating, being promiscuous or starting fights).

The reason why so much emphasis is placed on containing what we feel in psychodynamic work is because Freud believed that there was a destructive drive in human nature that had to be managed. He had witnessed two world wars and spent the last year of his life in London (fleeing from the Nazis). He ended his 1930 book *Civilization and Its Discontents* with the following observation: 'Eternal Eros will make an effort to assert himself in the struggle with his immortal adversary. But who can foresee with what success and with what result' (p. 340).

Of course Eros refers to our drive towards life and reparation, whereas Thanatos is a human drive towards destruction. According to Freud we have an inbuilt tendency towards carelessness, irregularity and unreliability and this explains why we value beauty, cleanliness and order, because they represent countervailing forces against disintegration and destructiveness. According to this perspective, all of us (to a greater or lesser extent) will experience a tension between parts of us that are more life affirming and aspects of us that are more destructive. This observation of human destructiveness changed Freud's view of therapy. It was now important, he said, to manage and contain emotional urges, rather than release them all via cathartic therapy. The aim of therapy was now to strengthen the ego or 'wise mind'.

According to this approach, our clients will also feel a tension and may be very alarmed by their own destructive tendencies and need help harnessing the sides of themselves they feel are more reparative and protective. As a mental health worker, you might, for example, be your client's first experience of someone who wants to help them to develop and strengthen their capacities for repair, but a client's feelings towards you may be strongly influenced by their past experience of carers – what is called transference. It involves asking yourself whom you might represent or be for someone in their internal world. Similarly, you need to ask who they are for you and this might be affected by who they are, but also by your own past experiences. This is the counter-transference. Does a client, for example, remind you of a loved sister and does this affect how you relate to them? Do you have strong transference reactions to people you work with (consultant psychiatrists or clinical psychologists, for example), do you attribute certain qualities to people that might say more about you than about them?

Psychodynamic approaches to self-reflection ask us to develop an internal observer who can watch the play of our minds like we might watch the play of children, without forcing their attention (Meltzer 1990). Although there are major differences between psychodynamic approaches and mindfulness practice, there are important commonalities too. Mindfulness also asks us to watch the play of the mind (In acceptance and commitment therapy (ACT) this is likened to watching our thoughts placed on leaves floating down stream (Baer 2006).) Both approaches ask us to withstand the feelings and thoughts that pulse through us and to develop compassionate observational capacities. Psychodynamic approaches do not call for a punitive internal observer, because it is recognized that we all move between different states of mind and feeling in relation to ourselves and to others.

The ego and defence mechanisms

There are, according to psychoanalysis, many anxieties that besiege us through life (as children, adolescents, lovers, etc.) and, although psychoanalytical writers are interested in a person's capacity to love, care, nurture and be creative, they nevertheless focus on the defences and pain which, to them, are part of being human. They suggest that we find it hard to bear pain and we naturally try to move away from it. It is for this reason that psychodynamic practitioners are interested in the defence mechanisms that we may habitually and unconsciously use. Individuals develop defences against discomfort, anxiety, pain, threats. Although some defences are necessary and facilitate the completion of a task, many are pathological and adversely affect our capacity to care. We might oscillate between different states of mind in relation to the world (for example, paranoid versus trusting) and this approach asks us to think about our way of relating to the world and about our defences when we feel particularly anxious.

Reflective Exercise 2.6

Defences and unconscious communication

Read the descriptions of some defences and some forms of unconscious communication given in Box 2.1. Now identify the defences or unconscious communication that might be operating in the extracts below and how you might deal with them (see Jacobs 2000):

- Alan qualifies everything you say with, 'Yes, but what about'.
- An adolescent boy is savagely attacked by a gang, but reports no memory of it.
- A young man has previously told you that he is worried about his partner's commitment to him, but now says that he could not wish for a more loyal partner.
- Betty tells you that she feels much better now after the last week when you began to touch on powerful feelings of loss.
- Charlie tells you of a huge row with his girlfriend after your one-to-one session with him.
- Doris tells you how helpful and understanding you are compared with all of your colleagues.
- Eddie says he can't get upset at his father's death, because he had such a good innings.
- You go to work feeling quite calm, but when you meet a colleague in crisis, they tell you that your work on the previous shift is being questioned and you end up feeling troubled and derailed.
- Fiona tells you that you are looking old and tired now, despite being similar in age to her and having helped her a lot.
- A client starts to use your dialect and vocabulary and reports that you are so alike. What does it make you feel?

(Some of the above extracts are taken from Jacobs (2000, p. 133).)

Box 2.1

Forms of defences and unconscious communication

- Repression – feelings and thoughts are almost completely forgotten and can come back in a disguised form.
- Denial – push a thought or feeling out of conscious awareness and resist an interpretation that brings it back to awareness.
- Splitting – idealize one person, denigrate another or vacillate between hating and loving the same person.
- Projection – we locate our uncomfortable feelings in another (we see them as envious, for example, rather than acknowledge that we feel it, or we might accuse them of being angry when it is what we feel).

- Projective identification – is a process whereby we treat someone else as if they represent a part of us (as with projection). This can nudge the other into behaving and feeling like us (they might start to feel envious and angry). Projective identification is therefore a process by which someone can feel what belongs to someone else, and perhaps act on it. It is a process of de-differentiation and self/other confusion/merger, yet it can also be used as a clue to what someone else is feeling (depressed, adolescent, de-skilled, excited and so on).

- Envy – another's achievement makes us feel deprived, cheated or lacking and we spoil the success or professional expertise of the other.

- Acting out – is a process whereby our unprocessed feelings or thoughts about something are discharged or expressed indirectly (via cutting or drinking, for example).

- Regression – is the process whereby we return to more child-like states of mind and feeling. If I want to evade adult responsibility, I might inhabit the world of a latency child or reckless adolescent.

- Rationalization – is the process whereby we account for something with a rational explanation that minimizes or denies what we feel.

- Displacement – is a process whereby we redirect our feelings about, for example, our family dynamics to another setting, for example work and berate our work colleagues for faults that might belong to our siblings or parents.

- Identification – involves unconsciously identifying with somebody in an adhesive way.

- Transference – is a process whereby we treat someone as if they were like someone else we know/knew (often, but not exclusively, one's early carers). For example, feelings of protectiveness, need and/or suspicion might be stirred up if a colleague, client or helper unconsciously reminds us of other significant people in our lives. Our feelings about our carers/parents, for example, can be transferred onto people in positions of power or care.

- Counter-transference – is our response to the transference reactions to us, but it also refers to the way in which our own early life affects the way we relate to our clients.

- Containment – is a process whereby we can receive emotional communications and not react or retaliate, but instead think through what the other person makes us feel and what this emotional exchange might mean or tell us. If we are being screamed at, provoked or exposed to another's unbearable pain, it can be very difficult to be containing and hold the feelings pushed into us, but this is central to mental health work. It is also crucially important for the developing child, who needs his/her parent to be able to hold the powerful feelings that he/she cannot yet manage to hold him/herself.

Psychodynamic approaches to care ask us to be aware of the dynamics that might be operating between us, particularly when we are anxious. They ask us to develop skills in emotional literacy so that we can read what emotional exchange might be taking place and know when we are subject to or responsible for a strong projection or projective identification. What we feel becomes a cue to understanding what someone else might feel, but it is only a cue or hint, it does not make us omnipotent readers of minds or hearts.

History repeats itself

Psychodynamic approaches to understanding mental health problems look to the past and present to do so. Our blueprint for relating to ourselves and to others is, according to this therapy, laid down in childhood. Freud (1923) said that 'living means the same as being loved' (p. 400) and psychodynamic practitioners are interested in whether, as children, clients felt loved or, for example, mocked, depended on or abused in order to understand their present difficulties. We all, according to this approach, fear separation (as children and adults) and need our anxieties to be soothed and contained by our carers. If our carers never did this we might not have had the chance to develop self-soothing behaviours that are reparative and instead turn to substitutive objects (drugs or food, for example) in order to assuage 'nameless dread' (Bion 1970).

Although there are differences between attachment theory and psychodynamic approaches, they both maintain that our early attachment patterns (secure, insecure, disorganized – see Hopkins 1990) are often repeated in later life and that without understanding the past we cannot understand the present. However, our early life is also likened to a prehistoric city that we need to excavate in order to see what traces of it remain.

Reflective Exercise 2.7

Genograms

One way to begin to think about the effect of the past on the present is to make a genogram. The genogram charts three generations and includes names, dates of birth, ages and genders. It can be used to look at intergenerational patterns. You might want to look at attachment patterns or the place of religion, sexuality or marriage and children in your family's life. If you haven't done this before, you might find it quite powerful. You can download templates for doing a genogram from the internet, with an explanation of the common set of symbols often used (for example an overly close relationship is depicted by three parallel lines between two members of your family). You could also look at the words that you circled as representing you in Exercise 2.1 to see which ones describe particular family members.

Healer, heal thyself

Cooper (2007) argues that 'in order to do mental health work well, we must be prepared to feel disturbed and distressed ourselves, at least some of the time. If we don't or can't, then surely we are not in true emotional contact with the very aspect of matters that needs our attention' (p. 576). Wilkin (2003) also states that we have to accept that we are as susceptible to being emotionally wounded as any other is and that, if we feel particularly emotionally fragile, we need to attend to our own wounds first (via supervision, therapy or time out). Indeed the new NMC competencies for mental health demand that practitioners:

value the importance of having an awareness of their own mental health and
well-being and the need to engage in reflection and supervision to explore the
emotional impact on self of working in mental health.

(Domain 1:4 and Domain 2:1)

Most psychodynamic trainings will require their trainees to be in therapy in order to address their own blind spots, defences and history. Cooper (2007) explains that therapeutic communities assume that 'everyone has ill or disturbed parts to them'. Hence staff have usually had therapy and 'continue to explore and value contact with their "disturbed" aspects because it is through understanding of these processes in themselves that they can be of help to others' (p. 570).

As with humanist psychology, this acknowledgement that we all have our internal battles, demons, fantasies and so on has a democratizing, normalizing effect, because we are not seen as wholly different from the people who seek our help. Ghaffari and Caparrotta (2004) argue that you have to be ill enough to need psychodynamic therapy, but well enough to withstand it. That is, you need to be able to make sure that you are ready to look at ghosts from the past and at yourself deeply. Some students are nervous about using this approach and opening the proverbial Pandora's box (one might ask whether it is already open for many of our clients). Interestingly the NMC competencies do not advise that you avoid distress and the disclosure of that which might be painful:

Mental health nurses must be sensitive to, and take account of, the impact of abuse
and trauma on peoples' well-being and the development of mental health
problems. Use interpersonal skills and make interventions that help people to
disclose and discuss their experiences as part of their recovery.

(Domain 4.1)

This work has to be done with sensitivity and compassion. Indeed Bettelheim (1982) referred to the soul or psyche as a bird or butterfly which one must approach with care in order not to crush it. You cannot start to work psychodynamically with clients without training or supervision, but you can use some of the ideas in order to think about how early traumas are often repeated and affect a person's self-esteem and capacity to be in relationships. You can also use these ideas to understand why you or a client might use a particular defence (they might not be able to bear their pain and scream it out at you, for example as in projection). The therapeutic relationship itself models how relationships can be robust, reliable and reparative. If it is successful it can be internalized and offset the internal images of relationships that are only bad, for example embittered, fractious or neglectful.

This approach points to the complexity of emotional life. If you try to learn from it, it might help you to attune to yourself and/or to your clients more, but it should not be used to force interpretations on people or to come to premature case formulations. By working through the following section you may be able to consolidate this section on psychodynamic practice.

Malan's two triangles

Malan (2002) introduces us to two tools to work with when using a psychodynamic approach. The 'triangle of conflict' illustrates a relationship between a hidden feeling or impulse, a corresponding anxiety and a defence against the anxiety. The second 'triangle of person' describes three people to whom the triangle of conflict might apply. These are people in one's current life, people in one's past and the person of the therapist or mental health worker. Interpretations are needed that link two or more points on the triangle. For example, I might have hidden feelings of grief or anger towards my parents (who neglected me as a child), which can be discerned in my current life (with my partner who I fear will abandon me), and in my relationship with my therapist (who I can't trust). This hidden feeling (grief, dread, anger) might make me anxious and I might use one of the above defences (denial or displacement, for example) in order to cope with the anxiety. If an interpretation is given at the right time about these links, I might see it at work in my current life and be able to change some aspects of it. But we have to know when we or others can bear to be in touch with feelings that might be deeply hidden and the therapeutic relationship is central to making this safe.

Malan (2002) argues that successful interpretations deepen the rapport between people and they can feel like symbolic love. However, Malan says that we should first look at the link between a defence (denial or displacement) in response to an anxiety and not go straight for an interpretation of hidden feeling. That is, as Bettelheim (1982) said, we need to approach the psyche with care. Malan also says that ideally we should also first explore links between a person's current life and past and not immediately make links between their past relationships and their relationships to helpers. Malan (2002) says that 'much of a therapist's skill consists of knowing which parts of a triangle to include in his interpretations at any given moment' (p. 91). Although you might not have been trained to use this approach directly with your clients, you can think about the following questions and see if it is an approach that helps you to understand yourself and is a good explanatory model for the genesis of mental health problems.

First triangle of person

1. Think of a client, person you know or think of yourself.

2. Tell a little about the types of relationship this person or you had as a child. How do you think they/you felt (secure, loved, humiliated, invisible, abused, neglected, manipulated). Were the relationships negative or positive?

3. Look at this person's/your own present life and describe the kinds of relationship that they/you have had in the recent past. Were they positive or negative? Which ones were significant? How did they/you behave and feel in them?

4. Can you see any links between the past and the recent past/present? Are there any patterns? Is this person/you mostly aware of them? If they/you are aware of them and want to change them, why can't you/they? Are there any positive aspects to their/your past relationships that are repeated in the present?

5. What is their relationship with you like (as a helper – see the idea of transference)? How do think that they see you (friend, enemy, mother, father, erotic partner)? What is your relationship like with people in authority/helping positions (look at your own transference)? How do you feel with your clients (see the idea of counter-transference)?

Second triangle of conflict/defence

1. What strong feelings or impulses do they/you have in relation to a significant other (heartache, love, longing, dread, envy, lust, fears of abandonment, excitement, tension, greed, anger)?

2. Do these feelings/impulses make them/you feel anxious?

3. What are their/your coping mechanisms/defences in the face of these feelings/impulses?

4. What anxiety/hidden feeling are they/you trying to avoid feeling by using these defences?

5. Are they/you aware of the defences that are used to cope in the world?

6. Are the defences that they use now similar to ones that might have been used in the past? Are they/you aware of this?

Take a simple example. Sam hates her mum for abandoning her (hidden feeling), but this feeling makes her feel very anxious and she defensively idealizes her relationship with her mother in order to stay away from the anxiety it causes. In her current relationship with her boyfriend, she is unhappy, but denies it to herself, because the thought of loss and abandonment is too threatening. She fears that her mental health worker does not really like her and she is very wary of showing how precarious and vulnerable she feels. What is the link between her past and present? How might she get in touch with her hidden feelings? What is her transference likely to be like? What counter-transference response might a mental health worker have?

These triangles are tools with which you can explore whether your current conflicts or dynamics are related to past events and feelings. They are guides for making that which might be habitual, repeated or unconscious more understandable and therefore changeable. They are aids and you can, of course, look at them and use them in order to think about who you are now. However, psychodynamic work takes place in the context of a live relationship with someone who is trained to know when it is safe to offer interpretations and explore links and when it is important to just sit and share someone's grief, for example (Malan 2002).

Section 4: philosophies of care – cognitive behavioural therapy

The same principle that has been adopted in Sections 1–3 continues here. That is, it is important to apply the principles of CBT to ourselves before we try to help someone else to use them. This will increase our understanding of what it is like for our clients. More specifically, for the purpose of this chapter we want to see what CBT tells us about the therapeutic use of self and how it can be used for reflective practice.

As with humanistic therapy and psychodynamic therapy, UCL has produced CORE national CBT competencies (Roth and Pilling 2011) and you can also look at the national Improving Access to Psychological Therapies (IAPT) initiative, which in its first phase has funded and rolled out CBT treatment on a widespread scale. This section will only introduce you to some basic reflexive tools that are commonly used in this approach, because, given the ubiquity of CBT, it is assumed that you might be more familiar with its philosophy and technique than you might be with the other two approaches that we have just discussed.

Like all other therapies, CBT relies on the practitioner being empathically skilled and able to develop therapeutic rapport. Unlike humanistic and psychodynamic practice, however, it is very structured and directive. Assessment is designed to lead to a case formulation and treatment targets which are directed towards cognitive and behavioural change. The case formulation template in Figure 2.1 shows you how an overall case might be conceptualized. Cognitive therapists might not work with a longitudinal formulation (as depicted in the figure), but, even if they do not work with the distant past, understanding a sequence of events and thoughts, feelings and behaviour in a client's past will nevertheless help them to see how a current problem has occurred and is being maintained. The CBT approach involves working with the way in which certain types of negative thinking are affecting how someone feels and behaves. Do you know what your own habitual negative thinking biases might be? Keep a simple thought diary for a few days and look at the link between an Antecedent or situation, a Belief and a Consequence (the ABC model – Table 2.4).

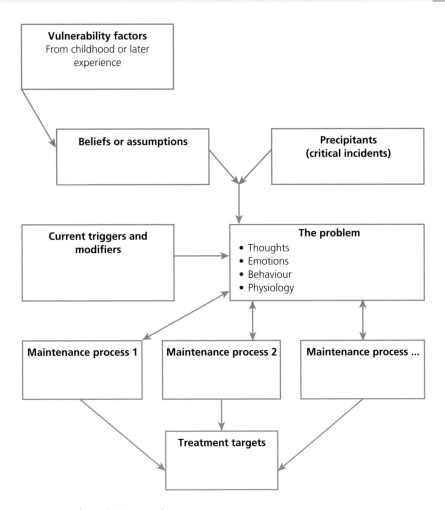

Figure 2.1 Case formulation template.

Table 2.4 The ABC model

	Antecedent event	Belief thought	Consequence
Monday	My colleague did not say hello to me yesterday morning	She does not like or respect me	I am not replying to her emails and we are both angry
Tuesday			
Wednesday			
Thursday			
Friday			

You can then develop this and keep a thought record which details a:

- Situation (as above)

- Mood (0–100) – (depressed 80/100)

- Hot, emotionally charged thought (as above)
  - Evidence for (She walked straight past me)
  - Evidence against (She is extremely busy and didn't see me)
- Alternative thought (She does respect and like me, I am being over-sensitive)
- Mood (0–100) – relaxed, not so depressed (40/100).

These thought diaries are very easy to keep and they could give you insight into common thinking patterns that you deploy. There are many good introductory textbooks (see Westbrook *et al.* 2007) that you can use in order to practise these thought diaries, activity schedules and behavioural experiments. Once you have looked at the link between your own thoughts and feelings, you can look at how they affect your behaviour. You can use the hot cross bun or cycle shown in Figure 2.2 to help you look at this. In the cycle in Figure 2.2 we see the way in which a negative thought jeopardizes a practitioner's training. Can you think of a problematic situation or behaviour that you might have similarly become stuck in? By finding out which of our behaviours are maintaining our problems, we can then target them as areas for treatment. For example if I stop giving case presentations, because I think I will look weak if I'm nervous, I do not give myself the chance to disconfirm the power of the thought, especially if I've stopped going to clinical supervision altogether.

I might have a dysfunctional assumption that states that 'You must never show frailty' and it might be a rule for living that I am completely unaware is dominating my life. It may be related to core beliefs I've developed in childhood ('I am unlovable'). But perhaps I don't need to dig down that far in order to change a present, incapacitating problem. If I try to change the negative thoughts, this alone might change my behaviour and consequently shift my self-experience.

In order to change your thoughts and behaviours, you need to be understanding, forgiving and not berate yourself for your failures or argue incessantly with yourself.

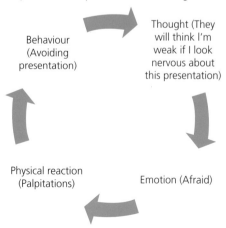

Figure 2.2 The hot cross bun or cycle.

The generic counselling and communication skills that are the core base for our other two psychological approaches are central here too. However, what is central to a therapeutic use of self in CBT is the ability to ask questions in a Socratic manner:

> Socrates, a philosopher living in Athens about 400BC ... spent his time in the marketplace encouraging the young men of Athens to question the truth of popular opinion. His unique approach was using questions to help his students reach a conclusion without directly instructing them. A Socratic question was one which the student had the ability to answer – although he might not realise it yet.

> (Westbrook et al. 2007, p. 90)

In CBT, Westbrook *et al.* similarly argue that questions are designed to help clients to review their own thoughts, feelings and behaviour from different perspectives and draw different conclusions about themselves. Imagine that you say to me that you feel worthless and I say 'That's stupid'. How helpful is that? If I argue with you, 'You are training to be a professional, you have qualifications' am I close to or far from your experience? If, rather than trying to argue with you, I try to gently shift your perspective (in time, place or person) I might convey patience and empathy, but also let you explore the truth of the thought. I might say 'Have you always thought that? Do you think you always will?' or 'What would your friends say if they heard you say this?' or 'What other images do you have of yourself'? This is an attempt to help someone to find some distance from a negative automatic thought and be able to evaluate the evidence for and against it. It also helps people to see that thoughts are not necessarily facts, but perspectives that can be changed.

Socratic questioning is not, however, unguided curiosity. It is hypothesis-led and guided by a formulation (Westbrook *et al.* 2007, p.103) leading to a treatment focus for the presenting problem. Moreover, Socratic questions are not always appropriate (in information gathering, for example, direct questions might be needed). Padesky (1993) referred to Socratic questioning as a form of guided discovery, rather than didactic lecturing or a forced attempt to change minds. In psychodynamic practice there is a similar emphasis on letting clients find their own interpretations. These will be the most powerful 'light bulb' moments when someone feels the realization about some aspect of themselves from deeply within, rather than as a message delivered to them externally. For example, you might have a clear hypothesis derived from a CBT case formulation about how a present problem is being maintained, but your role is to help the client to discover it for themselves and to become interested in their own minds as they do so.

Developing psychological mindedness is central to the therapeutic use of self in all of the therapies so far described. It refers to a curious, compassionate and robust observation of who we are and how we relate to others. It cannot all be taught in programmatic ways, but it might be possible to create conditions that facilitate it.

Conclusion: fellow feeling and self-care

This chapter has discussed what a therapeutic use of self involves. It is based on the idea of using the self as a healing agent by virtue of the manner in which we form and end relationships, as well as by virtue of the therapeutic techniques that we might use. Indeed the former is the bedrock for the latter. It has been shown that using the self as a therapeutic tool requires self-reflection, and this chapter has introduced you to some of the ways in which reflective practice might be conceptualized and practised in three major schools of psychology (which form the foundation for many contemporary therapies). The chapter did not aim to provide an in-depth or comprehensive account of these schools of psychology. What has been provided is necessarily a broad overview to give you a flavour of particular approaches and how you might use them to develop your own reflective and therapeutic skills.

We have seen the way in which many authors are concerned about whether contemporary mental health nursing is becoming more technical and less relational. There are debates about whether certain therapeutic approaches prioritize a prescribed set of techniques at the cost of developing therapeutic rapport and trust. The UK IAPT initiative has been both welcomed and criticized because of its emphasis on a nationally standardized and manualized way of doing therapy (House and Lowenthal 2008). This initiative, however, is informed by evidence (although as we saw from CORE what counts as contributing to evidence is a contested domain). We have also discussed the difficulty of isolating the variables that constitute a therapeutic use of self (good listening and responding, attunement, emotional literacy, and so on) and of measuring them. Nevertheless, there are measures for emotional intelligence (for example, Bar-On 2000), the Working Alliance Inventory (Horvath 2001), and so on, and we know that the therapeutic relationship is a major contributor to therapeutic outcomes (see CORE).

The aim of this chapter has not been to train you in evidence-based practice (see Chapter 6), but to provide you with self-reflective ideas and tools with which you can work. The more we are able to attune to the different tempos, thoughts and feelings that make up who we are, the more we will hopefully be able to attune to the plethora of voices, moods and rhythms of the people we work with. Freshwater and Stickley (2004) remind us that Perls said that 'one sigh may be communicating a lifetime of emotions. It is the emotionally intelligent practitioner that hears that sigh, makes eye contact, communicates understanding and demonstrates human care' (Perls 1973 cited in Freshwater and Stickley 2004, p. 92). Following this, there are many techniques that could be deployed to work with a person's lifetime of emotions, but first it is necessary to find a place in yourself where their sighs can be received, contained and metabolized. Moreover, you will first need a space in which you can listen to your own lifetime of emotions and also give yourself this necessary time and care. It is for this reason that your mental health training will hopefully enable a personal transformation for you that is in itself therapeutic. This does not mean that your training is itself a therapy and it should not be confused with one, but it might provide space for you to gently and possibly very privately review who you are and why you have chosen to join the mental health profession.

References

Abraham A (2011) *Care and Compassion? Report of the Health Service Ombudsman on Ten Investigations into NHS Care of Older People.* London: HMSO.

Altschul A (1997) A personal view of psychiatric nursing, in Tilley S (ed.) *The Mental Health Nurse: Views of Practice and Education.* Oxford: Blackwell Science.

Aslan M, Smith M (2007) *Thrive.* Coventry: Clifford Press.

Baer RA (2006) *Mindfulness-Based Treatment Approaches: Clinician's Guide to Evidence Base and Applications.* London: Academic Press.

Barker P (1999)*The Philosophy and Practice of Psychiatric Nursing.* Edinburgh: Churchill Livingstone.

Barker P (2003) *Handbook of Psychiatric and Mental Health Nursing: The Craft of Caring.* London: Hodder Arnold.

Bar-On R (2000) *The Handbook of Emotional Intelligence.* New York, NY: Jossey-Bass.

Berk L, Macneill C, Castke D, Berk M (2008) The importance of the treatment alliance in bipolar disorder, in Gleeson JFM, Killackey E, Krstev H (eds) *Psychotherapies for the Psychoses: Theoretical, Cultural and Clinical Integration.* New York, NY: Routledge/Taylor and Francis.

Bettelheim B (1982) *Freud and Man's Soul.* London: Penguin.

Bion W (1970) *Attention and Interpretation.* London: Karnac Books.

Brown L (1993) (ed.) *The New Shorter Oxford English Dictionary (1993): Thumb Index Edition.* Oxford: Oxford University Press.

Brown J (2006) *A Psychosocial Exploration of Love and Intimacy.* Basingstoke: Palgrave.

Carper BA (1978) Fundamental patterns of knowing in nursing. *Advances in Nursing Science* **1**(1), 13–23.

Casement P (1985) *On Learning from the Patient.* London: Brunner-Routledge.

Cooper A (2003) Supervision in primary care: support or persecution? in Burton J, Launer J (eds) *Supervision and Support in Primary Care.* Abingdon: Radcliffe Medical Press.

Cooper A (2007) Social work with adults with mental health problems, in Wilson K, Ruch G, Lymbery M, Cooper A (eds) *Social Work: An Introduction to Contemporary Practice.* Harlow: Pearson Longman.

Craib I (1994) *The Importance of Disappointment.* London: Routledge.

Davies T (1997) *Humanism.* London: Routledge.

Department of Health (2011) *No Health Without Mental Health: A Cross-Governmental Mental Health Outcomes Strategy for People of All Ages.* London: DH.

Egan G (2010) *The Skilled Helper: A Systematic Approach to Effective Helping, 2nd edn.* Minnesota, MI: Brooks/Cole.

Fonagy P, Gyorgy G, Elliot L, Target M (2007) *Affect Regulation, Mentalisation and the Development of Self.* London: Karnac Books.

Freshwater D (2004) Emotional intelligence: developing emotionally literate training in mental health. *Mental Health Practice* **8**(4), 91–8.

Freshwater D, Stickley T (2004) The heart of the art: emotional intelligence in nurse education. *Nursing Inquiry* **11**(2), 91–8.

Freshwater D, Stickley T (2006) The art of listening in the therapeutic relationship. *Mental Health Practice* **9**(5), 12–18.

Freshwater D, Stickley T (2009) The concept of space in the context of the therapeutic relationship. *Mental Health Practice* **12**(6), 91–8.

Freud S (1923) *The Ego and the Id*. London: Penguin (The Penguin Freud Library, Vol. 11, 1991).

Freud S (1930) *Civilisation and Its Discontents*. London: Pelican (The Penguin Freud Library, Vol. 12, 1985).

Fromm E (1986) *For the Love of Life*. New York, NY: Free Press.

Fromm E (1988) *On Being Human*. New York, NY: Continuum.

Fromm E (1994) *The Art of Listening*. London: Constable

Furedi F (2003) *Therapy Culture: Cultivating Vulnerability in an Uncertain Age*. London: Routledge.

Ghaffari K, Caparrotta L (2004) *The Function of Assessment within Psychological Therapies: A Psychodynamic View*. London: Karnac Books.

Gibbs G (1988) *Learning by Doing: A Guide to Teaching and Learning Methods*. London: Further Education Unit.

Goleman D (1995) *Emotional Intelligence*. New York, NY: Bantam.

Heron D (1993) *Group Facilitation: Theory and Models for Practice*. East Brunswick, NJ: Nichols Publishing.

Hopkins J (1990) The observed infant of attachment theory. *British Journal of Psychotherapy* **6**(4), 460–70.

Hopkinson JB, Brown JC, Okamoto I, Addington-Hall JM (2011) The effectiveness of family intervention for the management of symptoms and other health-related problems in people affected by cancer: a systematic literature search and narrative review. *Journal of Symptom and Pain Management* **43**, 111–42.

Horvath AO (2001) Psychotherapy: theory, research, practice and training. *American Psychological Association* **38**(4), 365–72.

House R, Lowenthal D (2008) *Against and For CBT: Towards Constructive Dialogue*. Ross-on-Wye: PCCS Books.

Jacobs M (2000) *Swift to Hear: Facilitating Skills in Listening and Responding*, 2nd edn. London: SPCK.

Johns C (2004) *Becoming a Reflective Practitioner*, 2nd edn. Oxford: Blackwell Publishing.

Kabat-Zinn J (2005) *Full Catastrophe Living: Using the Wisdom of Your Body and Mind to Face Stress, Pain, and Illness*. New York, NY: Delta Trade Paperbacks.

Karver M, Shirk S, Handelsman JB, Fields S, Crisp H, Gudmendsen G, McMakin D (2008) Relationship processes in youth psychotherapy: Measuring alliance, alliance-building behaviours, and client involvement. *Journal of Emotional and Behavioural Disorders* **16**(1), 15–28.

Keen T, Lakeman R (2003) Collaboration with patients and families, in Barker P (ed.) *Handbook of Psychiatric and Mental Health Nursing: The Craft of Caring*. London: Hodder Arnold.

Klein M (1957) *Envy and Gratitude*. London: Virago (1988).

Lemma A, Roth AD, Pilling S (2011) *The Competences Required to Deliver Effective Psychoanalytic/Psychodynamic Therapy*. Online: www.ucl.ac.uk/CORE (accessed November 2011).

Luft J, Ingham H (1955) *The Johari Window: A Graphic Model of Interpersonal Awareness*. Proceedings of the Western Training Laboratory in Group Development. Los Angeles, CA: UCLA.

Mahaffey BA, Lewis MS (2008) Therapeutic alliance directions in marriage, couple, and family counselling, in Walz GR, Bleuer JC, Yep RK, Alexandria VA (eds) *Compelling Counselling Interventions*. Alexandria, VA: American Counselling Association, pp. 59–69.

Malan D (2002) *Individual Psychotherapy and the Science of Psychodynamics,* 2nd edn. London: Arnold.

Maslow A (1962) *Toward a New Psychology of Being.* New York, NY: D Van Nostrand Co.

McDougall J (1991) *Theatres of the Mind*. London: Free Association Books.

Mearns D, Thorn B (2007) *Person-Centred Counselling in Action,* 2nd edn. London: Sage.

Meltzer D (1990) *The Psychoanalytical Process*. Strathtay: Clunie Press.

Mezirow J (1981) A critical theory of adult learning and education. *Adult Education* **32**, 3–23.

NMC (2010) *Standards for Pre-Registration Nursing Education*. London: Nursing and Midwifery Council.

Orbach S (1999) *Towards Emotional Literacy*. London: Virago.

O'Shaughnessy E (1994) What is a clinical fact? *International Journal of Psycho-Analysis* **75**(5/6), 939–49.

Padesky C (1993) *Socratic Questioning: Changing Minds or Guiding Discovery?* Keynote address delivered at European Association for Behavioural and Cognitive Therapies conference, London.

Papastavrou E, Eftstathiou G, Charamalambous A (2011) Nurses' and patients' perceptions of caring behaviours: quantitative systematic review of comparative studies. *Journal of Advanced Nursing* **67**(6), 1191–205.

Peplau H (1952, 1988) *Interpersonal Relations in Nursing*. Basingstoke: Macmillan.

Perls F (1973) *The Gestalt Approach and Eye Witness to Therapy*. Palo Alto, CA: Science and Behaviour Books.

Reynolds B (2003) Developing therapeutic one-to-one relationships, in Barker P (ed.) *Handbook of Psychiatric and Mental Health Nursing: The Craft of Caring*. London: Hodder Arnold.

Richards B, Brown J (2011) Media as drivers of the therapeutic trend? *Free Associations* **62**, 18–30.

Rippere V, Williams R (eds) (1985) *Wounded Healers*. London: John Wiley & Sons.

Roth AD, Pilling S (2011) *The Competences Required to Deliver Cognitive and Behavioural Therapy for People with Depression and Anxiety Disorders*. Online: www.ucl.ac.uk/CORE (accessed November 2011).

Roth AD, Hill A, Pilling S (2011) *The Competences Required to Deliver Effective Humanistic Psychological Therapies*. Online: www.ucl.ac.uk/CORE (accessed November 2011).

Sartre JP (1948) *Anti-Semite and Jew*. New York, NY: Schchen Books.

Schon D (1987) *Educating the Reflective Practitioner*. San Fransciso, CA: Jossey-Bass.

Schultz HJ (1986) In the name of life: a portrait through dialogue, in Fromm E (ed.) *For the Love of Life*. New York, NY: Free Press.

Shirk SR, Gudmundsen G, Kaplinski HC, McMakin DL (2008) Alliance and outcome in cognitive-behavioural therapy for adolescent depression. *Journal of Clinical Child and Adolescent Psychology* **37**(3), 631–9.

Smith P (1999) Theology of emotion. *Soundings: A Journal of Politics and Culture* **11**, 152–8.

Smythe EA (2004) Thinking. *Nurse Education Today* **24**, 326–32.

Stern D (1985) *The Interpersonal World of the Infant: A View from Psychoanalysis and Developmental Psychology*. New York, NY: Basic Books.

Street R Jr, Makoul G, Arora N, Epstein RM (2009) How does communication heal? Pathways linking clinician-patient communication to health outcomes. *Patient Education and Counselling* **74**(3), 295–301.

Symington N (1986) *The Analytic Experience*. London: Free Association Books.

von Esen L, Sjoden PO (1993) Perceived importance of caring behaviours to Swedish psychiatric inpatients and staff, with comparisons to somatically ill samples. *Research in Nursing and Health* **16**, 293–303.

Westbrook D, Kennerley H, Kirk J (2007) *An Introduction to Cognitive Behaviour Therapy: Skills and Applications*. London: Sage.

Wilkin P (2003) The craft of psychiatric-mental health nursing practice, in Barker P (ed.) *Handbook of Psychiatric and Mental Health Nursing: The Craft of Caring*. London: Hodder Arnold.

Yalom I (2001) *The Gift of Therapy: Reflections on Being a Therapist*. London: Piatkus.

Zeldin T (1995) *An Intimate History of Humanity*. London: Minerva.

CHAPTER THREE

Chris McLean, Bill Fulford and **Diane Carpenter**

Values-based practice

Learning outcomes

- Be able to articulate and critically reflect on your own personal values
- Be able to critically discuss the nature of professional values and how these may relate to personal values
- Be able to evaluate the importance of recognizing and working with the personal values of others
- Be able to identify the skills that you will need to develop for values-based mental health practice

What is values-based practice?

Values-based practice is an approach that recognizes that the values of both service users and ourselves are inescapable in health care. Our own personal values, our professional values and the values of the people we care for are all inextricably involved in every aspect of our clinical practice and decision-making. Health care professionals therefore need to develop skills and attitudes which enable them to recognize, work with, and respond to their own values and those of others.

Evidence-based medicine was first brought to prominence by Sackett and colleagues in the early 1990s and has been defined as 'the conscientious, explicit and judicious use of current best evidence in making decisions about the care of individual patients' (Sackett *et al.* 1996). Although proponents of evidence-based practice recognize the need for 'the integration of best research evidence with clinical expertise and patient values' (Sackett *et al.* 2000), the evidence-based practice movement does not itself provide an understanding of the skills and attitudes which are necessary to work with *values*. All decision-making requires that we attend to values as well as facts, and while evidence can tell us with varying degrees of certainty what outcomes may follow from certain interventions or treatment options, only the ability to understand and work with values can help us to understand which of these outcomes will be valued from the unique perspective of any one service user. In this regard, values-based practice can be seen as the sister (and complementary) framework to the evidenced-based practice movement. See also the *Values-Based Practice Reading Guide* produced by the University of Warwick (2010).

One of the main reasons that values are easily overlooked in decision-making is that, if they are not obviously conflicting, they are often presumed to be shared. Fulford gives examples such that choices between 'acting in a person's best interest' and valuing patient autonomy can often reveal conflicting value frameworks (2011, p. 976). An example might be making a decision about facilitating escorted leave for a patient detained under mental health legislation. Basing a decision upon ethical principles (closely linked to values) might require an intervention which would do good (beneficence), prevent harm (non-maleficence), be fair and equitable and respect the autonomy of the individual (see Beauchamp and Childress 2001). In applying these principles, it can be recognized that making judgements about what constitutes 'good' or 'harm' requires an appreciation of what is important to (the values of) the service user and others: the escorted leave would probably be facilitated if a risk assessment indicated it would be safe. However, if the ward were short staffed then a utilitarian approach to justice – promoting the greatest good for the greater number – may require valuing the benefits to the whole patient group more highly than the autonomy of one individual.

For this reason the ability to both recognize and respond to *differences* in values between ourselves and others is central to values-based practice. At the same time we should note that 'much of how we see ourselves is determined by what we value, and our values express who and what we are' (Mohr *et al.* 2001, p. 31). While in any given situation we have a tendency to presume that values are shared, our values are therefore also central to the way in which we see and construct ourselves as unique individuals. Although values can be shared, our values also define us as different from others, and if other people think and behave in ways which suggest their values are different from our own then it is easy to see them as somehow 'other' to ourselves. This construction of 'otherness', of seeing others as different from and separate from ourselves, can be identified as the first step towards stereotyping, prejudice and exclusion. It is therefore essential that we pay attention to our own and others' values in every situation, and not only when we see an immediately apparent problem or complexity. The links between these considerations and the issue of inclusion are discussed further in Chapter 5.

In mental health practice our understanding of service users can be influenced by this sense of 'otherness', and recent developments in service user involvement aim to foster new ways of thinking which contrast with the 'medical and therapeutic' models that have previously dominated health care. A values-based approach moves away from viewing mental health in terms of individual limitations and inabilities, and instead places its main emphasis on addressing the different barriers and obstacles that prevent people from participating fully in their own decision-making process. There is a need for ways of working which recognize service users as active members of the decision-making process, and this means that our own professional values as health care practitioners must be based on ensuring that the values of service users are the basis for our own decisions. This shift may challenge traditional personal and professional modes of thinking, and also highlights how organizational cultures and structures need to respond and change in order to accommodate new partnerships with service users.

Service users and their families continue to report that they often feel excluded from decision-making, care and treatment processes, and yet it is clear that decisions about an individual's care should be made as a team with the values of the individual service user at their centre. There is consistent evidence that mutually respectful collaborative alliances between professionals and patients are of central importance in determining the outcome of any therapeutic strategy, and Chapter 2 addressed this in detail. Values-based practice is therefore an approach to supporting clinical decision-making that highlights the skills and attitudes which are necessary for practitioners to realize the vision of the Department of Health (DH) that there should be 'No decision about me without me' (DH 2010b). The remainder of this chapter begins to address the practice skills which need to be developed in order to enable nurses and other mental health practitioners to negotiate care delivery through eliciting and responding to the individual values of service users.

To address the complexity of working with values, Fulford (2004) has developed a conceptual framework for values-based decision-making. Values-based practice may be considered as 'the theory and capabilities for effective decision making in health and social care that builds in a positive way on differences and diversity of values' (Fulford *et al.* 2012). Ten key principles have been identified as central to values-based practice (Box 3.1).

Woodbridge and Fulford (2004) note that putting these principles into practice requires gaining skills in four key areas. These are: (1) gaining a raised awareness of the values that are relevant in any particular situation; (2) reasoning with and about values; (3) knowledge of values; and (4) communication skills. Points 1–3 are addressed here, whilst Chapter 2 explores communication and relational skills in mental health practice. To become aware of the ways in which values are relevant in any particular situation requires that we are aware of ourselves and the influence of our own personal values in any situation. Our starting point as a vital pre-requisite for values-based practice is self-awareness.

Box 3.1

Fulford's 10 principles of values-based practice skills enable us to apply values-based practice in each interaction with service users

Practice skills

- Awareness: ensuring you are aware of the values that may play a part in a particular situation
- Reasoning: using values as part of your decision-making process to determine 'what is right'
- Knowledge: know about values and facts that are relevant to your situation
- Communication: using communication skills to resolve conflicts/complexity

Models of service delivery

- User-centred: considering the service user's values as the first priority in a given decision
- Multi-disciplinary: using a balance of perspectives to resolve conflicts

Values-based practice and evidence-based practice

- The 'two feet' principle: all decisions are based on facts and values; evidence-based practice and values-based practice therefore work together
- The 'squeaky wheel' principle: values should be involved in all situations and not just be noticed if there is a problem or complex decision to be taken
- Science and values: increasing scientific knowledge and evidence-based practice create choices in health care; this can lead to wider differences in values

Partnership

- Partnership: within values-based practice it is important that decisions are taken by service users working in partnership with providers of care

Adapted from: Fulford KWM (2004) Ten principles of values based medicine, in Radden J (2004) *The Philosophy of Psychiatry: A Companion.* New York, NY: Oxford University Press, pp. 206–34.

Self-awareness and personal values

We have noted that values are central to the way in which we define ourselves as individuals and consequently that our sense of who we are and our personal values are inextricably linked. To know who we are (and who we are being at any moment in time) is to be aware of our values. No one would deny that values are important, but discussing and working with values can soon become complicated. If you were to ask a range of different people to define values you would undoubtedly receive a range of answers (you may wish to experiment with this). In general though, values relate to our goals or aims, and what we think is worthwhile and what would constitute a 'good life' for us. Given that we all want different things and have different ideas about what constitutes a good life, our personal values will be different. Nonetheless our personal values can be defined as the standards against which we judge whether we are 'thriving' and living the life that we want to.

Reflective Exercise 3.1

Reflect on the following questions:

* What would constitute a 'good life' to you?
* Have your ideas about what you want out of life ever changed?
* Do you feel that you always live up to your personal values?
* What does this exercise tell you about your personal values?

Given the points made in the introduction to this chapter and perhaps taking account of your responses to the questions in Reflective Exercise 3.1, we can make the following observations about personal values.

* People have different ideas about what constitutes a 'good life' and therefore have different values.

* Personal values may change and develop. Our idea of what constitutes a good life will vary according to our age or health, and in relation to the life opportunities which are afforded to us.

* Personal values represent a goal or an ideal, and are not readily 'achieved'. We may easily recognize that an individual who values money will never have enough. Similarly, an individual who values care and compassion may never feel that they 'care' enough. In this sense, we never fully embody our values, but simply work towards achieving them.

* Personal values can evolve and can be chosen.

It is particularly important to note that our values are reflected in our behaviour, our choices and what we actually do. Our values represent the goals which we are seeking to achieve in life, and so by becoming aware of our behaviour and the choices which we make we can become aware of our true values. The objectivity this requires can be challenging given that we tend to want to see ourselves in a favourable light, and reflecting on our values while being honest with ourselves can take courage, maturity and integrity.

You may wish to think about the questions in Reflective Exercise 3.2 to help you to begin to clarify your own personal values.

Reflective Exercise 3.2

- Think of something which you have done or achieved in your personal life which you were proud of. Why were you proud?
- You may also want to think about something in your personal life which you regret not having done. Why did you regret this?

Answering these questions may help you to articulate what it is that you consider to be living a 'good life', and begin to help clarify your personal values. Hopefully, thinking about these questions will also have helped you to appreciate the ways in which peoples' values can be inferred from their behaviours.

Professional values

Caring is essentially an encounter between one person and another, and managing differences and tensions between our own personal values and the values of the people we care for is at the heart of values-based practice. However, as health care practitioners, we work with others not only as individuals with our own personal values, but also as professionals. While our personal values are intimately linked to who *we* are, it is our professional values that define the *practitioner* we are. This requires us to consider the nature of *professional* values in health care. Although this book is directed to meet the specific needs of mental health nurses, values-based practice demands the same core professional values of all health care practitioners. Currently roles in health care are developing rapidly, there is an increasing focus on inter-professional learning and the most recent standards for the education of nurses (Nursing and Midwifery Council (NMC) 2010) have emphasized that all nurses need to share the same core skills, attitudes and values. In this context it is appropriate to consider the values which underpin the practice of health care, rather than to narrowly consider the values of mental health nursing.

The National Health Service (NHS) constitution (DH 2010a) makes claims that health care in England will be founded upon the values of care, respect and compassion, but interpreting what these values actually mean is not straightforward. We take the view that health care is a 'practice' (MacIntyre 1985) in the sense that it is a co-operative activity which has its own standards of excellence, and which seeks to achieve particular goals. If the practice of health care is to be responsive to the personal values of others, the goal of health care may be characterized as being to ensure that the people we care for become more able to live a good life, or to see that they 'flourish' (Sellman 2011) or 'thrive'. Smith and Aslan develop the concept of 'thriving' in Chapter 9 in this volume, but the values of care, respect and compassion must therefore relate to the ways in which we help others to thrive.

We have already noted that all values are a standard of excellence, and that we all have unique personal values and our own personal ideas about what constitutes living a good life. Putting all of these points together allows us to recognize that these professional values of care and compassion may be seen as the standards against which we judge how well we help *others* to thrive, and the extent to which we respond to the values of service users.

The many ways in which mental health nurses may ensure that others 'thrive' is the subject of the remainder of this book, but we can see already that professional values are not straightforward. It is not immediately clear, for example, whether 'helping' or 'solving problems' could be characterized as ensuring that others thrive (what if they do not want 'help'?, or if our 'solutions' are not in accordance with what they see as a good life?). On the other hand, respect for the personal values of others demands that we demonstrate care and compassion (although we may have different views on what this means). From this, we may make the following observations about professional values.

- Our professional values define who we are as a practitioner.
- Professional values in health care must incorporate concepts of respect, care and compassion for the person.
- Health care practitioners may have different ideas about what constitutes 'thriving' or about how this may be ensured. Individual practitioners may therefore have different professional values.
- The way in which we may ensure that others thrive may vary in different contexts, and values are therefore contextual and situational.
- Professional values are criteria for excellence. None of us is perfect, and we may fail to live up to our values in every respect. Professional development, therefore, requires having secure professional values, being able to recognize when we are not behaving in accordance with these and being willing to work to develop the habits of thought which will enable us to behave consistently with our professional values.

A mental health nurse plays a key role in ensuring that others 'thrive' and, while they must possess professional values which are based on care and compassion, this is only the beginning of an understanding. 'Caring' can mean many things to different people or in different contexts and may be seen as (among other things) a practical activity; a virtue or character trait; an emotional response or as a type of relationship.

Try Reflective Exercise 3.3 to begin trying to clarify your own professional values, and what care and compassion may mean to you.

What Reflective Exercise 3.3 may have demonstrated to you is that professional values are difficult to define. Although professional values in nursing will be based on care and compassion, every nurse will develop their own ideas of what they mean and their own standards for excellence.

If you have considered what may be meant by care and compassion, it is also likely that you will have realized that mental health nursing will involve the use of your whole self as a person (including emotions and feelings). Chapters 2 and 4 provide examples of how to deepen your self-awareness in this respect. The above considerations also highlight that care and compassion are not part of a 'job', but are fundamentally a part of who you *are*. Caring in nursing practice has been described as something of a paradox given that nurses are 'required by one's job to do emotional work which needs to be felt spontaneously' (Chambliss 1996, p. 2). It may be seen, however, that this is only a paradox if you continue to think of nursing as something you do, rather than something you are. Something has motivated you to enter the profession of mental health nursing and this means that becoming a mental health nurse is (presumably) something which you value and consider to be part of a 'good life' for yourself. To act in accordance with this value is to accept that you need to consider and adopt professional values in order to become the nurse you want to be. It is a matter of your personal integrity to act in accordance with your own values, and it is this which will lead you to act consistently with your professional values.

Ultimately you must do all of this yourself. It is now many years since Florence Nightingale observed in relation to teaching nursing students that: 'I do not pretend to teach her how, I ask her to teach herself, and for this purpose I venture to give her some hints' (Nightingale 1860, p. 1). The aim of this chapter is to give such hints, and to introduce you to some of the essential skills which you will need if you are to develop into the practitioner who you wish to become.

Introducing a model for values-based enquiry

Having considered these preliminaries, we shall begin to explore a model which illustrates a way of thinking about how personal and professional values may be considered in relation to decision-making within health and social care so as to build on differences and diversity in values. The aims of the values-based enquiry model are to develop and maintain a focus on our own personal and professional values, and to recognize that if we are true to these values then our personal integrity itself will help us remain responsive to the values of others.

The model has been developed to help practitioners foster the development of a professional identity having the knowledge, skills, caring attitudes and courage to provide values-based care. This may be achieved through developing 'habits' of mind which are associated with demonstrating care and compassion, personal courage and intellectual rigour.

As a model for self-development, values-based practice aims to develop us as reflexive practitioners by challenging us to recognize dissonance between our values and our behaviours. Working through the values-based enquiry model can be an experiential process, although it is helpful to highlight that there are two distinct perspectives within the model.

A focus on the challenges and rewards of practice

The model presented provides a space to reflect and consider our personal and professional values and the way in which we consequently respond to the values of others. Through this process it is intended that we recognize the challenges and the rewards of nursing practice to provide motivation for further learning and development. You may wish to think about the questions in Reflective Exercise 3.4, which reflect the earlier exercise in relation to your *personal* values.

Reflective Exercise 3.4

- Think of something which you have done or achieved in an interaction with a service user which you were proud of. Why were you proud?
- You may also want to think about something in your professional life which you regret not having done. Why did you regret this?

Answering these questions may help you to articulate what you consider being a good mental health nurse is and so begin to help in clarifying your professional values.

Hopefully you will recognize that those moments in which you have been proud of yourself are immensely rewarding. Recognition of the rewards which you can experience through being the nurse who you wish to be can be a powerful motivator for further professional growth. The realization that we may have regrets about not being able to be the nurse we may wish to be also highlights one of the most difficult challenges in mental health nursing practice.

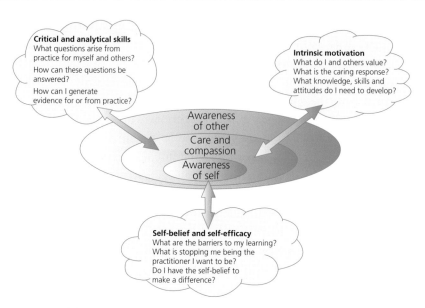

Figure 3.1 A model for values-based enquiry.

Reflection on practice and service user involvement

When we take a step back from a particular interaction with a service user, we may reflect on our practice in ways which may guide our future development. We can learn to develop habits of mind that encourage us to question how we could further ensure that our practice is responsive to the needs of others and that service users are always fully involved as partners in care. The above elements relate to the 'core' of the model and to the surrounding three sets of prompt questions respectively (Fig. 3.1).

The following sections will introduce and guide you through the use of this model for values-based practice.

Meet Iain: using the values-based model

In the sections that follow, we will use a case study to help you to work through the elements of the values-based model. In this way you will begin to gain an understanding of how the model may help you develop the skills that are necessary for values-based practice. The starting point of the model is self-awareness.

Self-awareness

Self-awareness (Fig. 3.2) not only means being aware of the values that help to define who we are as people, but also means having the ability to remain aware of how these values influence us in every moment. In this respect, self-awareness requires the ability

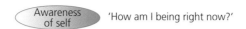

'How am I being right now?'

Figure 3.2 Starting to use the values-based model: self-awareness.

for 'reflection-in-action', which Christopher Johns describes as the 'constant monitoring of the self in the situation' (Johns and Freshwater 1998, p. 14). Self-awareness in any situation therefore means asking oneself 'How am I being right now?'

This part of the model, therefore, aims to encourage the 'constant monitoring of the self', which is central to reflection *in* action. Through asking ourselves 'How am I being right now?' we are enabled to:

- Develop awareness of our own personal values and beliefs

- Become aware of our own behaviour in each moment.

In the exercises related to Case Study 3.1 below, we want you to concentrate on a central concern to us in mental health care – how our personal values inform how we work in practice.

Case Study 3.1

Meeting Iain

Reading through the brief referral letter from Iain's general practitioner (GP) I was aware that I was meeting a recently relapsed heroin user, who in the view of the GP was an entrenched drug-seeking individual.

I was working within a small semi-rural community hospital where the drug service had the use of a small room to meet local people presenting with drug and alcohol problems. It was a difficult environment where I had concerns about maintaining client confidentiality because of the open nature of the general waiting area. Many of our service users would choose to travel to the nearest town for appointments and/or drug counselling rather than being seen attending at the local hospital.

My first meeting with Iain was to be in the general waiting area when I would invite him to come to our meeting room. On entering the waiting area I was immediately aware of a man sitting apart from the other service users and attracting some curiosity from others waiting in the area. He was obviously anxious, nervous and unable to sit still, and was clearly distressed. He was dressed in camouflage clothes and smelt strongly of patchouli oil, indeed looking and acting like an archetypal 'hippy' drug user.

Reflective Exercise 3.5

Take some time to reflect and ask yourself the following questions:

- If you were seeing Iain in the waiting area how would you go about clarifying your own thinking?
- What are your thoughts and feeling about Iain? How do these feelings relate to your own personal values?
- From the way this account is written, what values do you think are important for the nurse who is writing?

Mental health nurses bring to any encounter with a service user the values which they have attained through their previous life experiences. This cannot be helped and should not be apologized for – as we noted previously these values themselves are a part of who we are. Nonetheless, it is important to recognize that these values will mean that in meeting Iain, as in any other interaction, the nurse will experience an initial emotional response over which he or she has little control. True self-awareness means not only examining the reasons for these responses and the values which they reflect, but also having the ability to monitor ourselves within the situation so as to remain aware of them at the time. Self-awareness is, therefore, not only a foundational skill underpinning reflective practice, but is also essential in enabling us to understand and build therapeutic relationships with service users and their families (Burns and Bulman 2000). As Burnard (2002) notes, being self-aware allows us:

> *to select therapeutic interventions from a range of options so that the patient or client benefits more completely. If we are blind to ourselves we are also blind to our choices. We are blind, then, to caring and therapeutic choices.*

> *(p. 36)*

Recognizing professional values

Let us return to our case study of Iain and explore this further by looking at what may constitute a caring and compassionate response (Fig. 3.3). This requires us to ask ourselves what this may actually mean in any unique interaction with a service user.

Read the extract in the continuation of Case Study 3.1 below before considering the questions that follow.

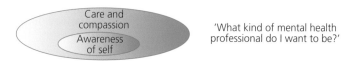

Figure 3.3 Being caring and compassionate.

Case Study 3.1

Continued

I built a therapeutic alliance immediately with Iain as his manner was gentle and quietly engaging. He told a story of using opiates when he lived in Glasgow as a young man and of stopping opiate use about 15 years previously when he had a serious motorcycle accident resulting in a three-month stay in Glasgow Royal Infirmary with several fractures to both lower legs and a further fracture to his cervical spine.

Following his recovery he had decided to move away and make a fresh start – he had subsequently married and had three children. He had continued to experience some pain in his lower back and self-medicated with home-grown cannabis.

Over the last six months the back pain had become worse with increasing poor mobility. He had visited his GP on several occasions requesting help for pain management; these visits had resulted in prescriptions for ibuprofen, which Iain felt was an inadequate response to his pain.

About three months previously, following several nights of poor sleep as a result of increasing pain, he had purchased street opiates and had continued using these intravenously in increasing amounts. His current reported daily use was between 0.75 and 1 g of opiates, costing him about £80 a day. He reported a low mood state and some suicidal ideation – but said he had not acted on these feelings because of the hurt this would cause to his wife and children.

Following the discovery of a very overdrawn credit card he had confessed his situation to his wife, who was saying that unless he sorted himself out immediately she was ending the relationship because of the potential impact the drug use would have on the children.

Reflective Exercise 3.6

- Can you see or comment on any value judgements that the nurse may be exhibiting in this extract?
- What would care and compassion mean in providing care to Iain in this situation?
- Are there any other professional values which are not being demonstrated that you think are an important part of being a good mental health nurse?
- What evidence do you need (or what questions may you ask) if you are to provide values-based care to Iain?

Working with values of others

The next stage of the model requires that we now consider how we may recognize and respond to the values of others (Fig. 3.4). Again, read the continuation of Iain's story below and then think about the questions which follow.

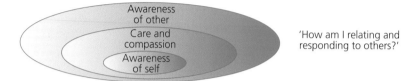

'How am I relating and responding to others?'

Figure 3.4   Recognizing and responding to the values of others.

Case Study 3.1

Continued

I have been working with Iain for about six months now and he is making excellent progress. We have been working closely with the pain clinic and he is stabilized on a reducing dose of methadone, dihydrocodeine and amitriptyline to manage his pain.

During our session today we focused on perceptions of pain and explored how positive thinking could be an important adjunct to managing Iain's chronic pain. As part of this we undertook some imagery work by exploring a situation where Iain would expect to feel pain. We first formed an active mental picture of the event that was about to happen. We built this picture by incorporating past experiences with the imagined situation and what Iain believed would happen. We then undertook an exploration of the factors that change the way he perceived pain and how pain could be viewed as more intense or less intense depending on the situation.

The exercise did not go well and I left the session feeling frustrated with Iain as he seemed 'stuck' with the belief that opiates were the only solution to control his pain.

Reflective Exercise 3.7

- What values do you think are important in Iain's decision-making process? Can you identify with any of these?
- How would you explain any perceived conflict or dissonance between Iain's values and those of the nurse?
- What would you do or say in order to find out more about the values that are important to Iain?

These questions highlight that identifying Iain's health needs will depend on how Iain himself defines his health. There is a danger that health professionals may define health narrowly as the absence of disease, and yet it is clear that the decisions that need to be made regarding Iain's care must be made with regard to his own values. Iain is presenting with multiple needs – social, physical and psychological – and to help him to thrive (or flourish) will require an understanding of his own values and priorities. Considering Iain's own values is essential for the nurse to support Iain with all of these presenting needs and in determining which problem(s) ought to be prioritized.

Considering the above questions may also have highlighted that responding to the values of others may first require that we enable service users to identify their own values system. If service users are not helped to clearly express their values and what is important to them, decision-making may be based on confusion or misunderstanding. Ultimately, both the nurse and Iain himself will need to be clear about their values if decisions about Iain's care are to be made without passing judgement and in the light of what is possible within the capabilities and resources of the health provider.

Reflecting on Iain's care

The above discussion highlights how in one sense the abilities to remain self-aware, to understand one's own professional values, and to clarify and respond to the values of others may be understood as skills which may be acquired. In gaining an appreciation of the skills involved it may help to concentrate on these aspects as discrete entities, and to break them down in the way that we have done in the exercises above.

Once we have acquired these skills however, the ability to respond to the values of others becomes simply a part of who we are. If we do hold values of care and compassion which relate to enabling others to thrive, then ensuring that our practice is values based becomes a matter of personal integrity. Responding to the values of others can become a matter of habit and a part of who we (or at least who our professional selves) are. In short, values-based practice is a matter of our character.

The model we present highlights that values-based practice requires three aspects of our character. First, it is important that we remind ourselves of our own intrinsic motivation to care and whether in any situation we have considered the question posed by Tschudin (2003) of what may constitute a caring response. Second, we may recognize that a commitment to evidence-based practice is important, and that questions will arise from our practice for which we can seek evidence to increase our understanding. Finally we may recognize that if we are, in fact, to be the practitioners that we wish to be then we need to consider whether we have the courage and personal efficacy which are necessary both for values-based practice and which our professional development require. The prompt questions within the model shown in Figure 3.1 are designed to help you to reflect on your own practice and learning in order to guide your development as a values-based practitioner.

The three sets of prompt questions within the model represent 'habits of mind', which we are seeking to develop as health professionals. It is intended that these prompt questions 'lead in' to questions relating to self-awareness and professional values, or may 'lead out' to guide further learning and development.

Reflective Exercise 3.8

Consider a recent significant episode in your own professional life.

- Asking yourself many of the questions in the model above may lead you to revisit questions we have previously considered. These may relate to how you recognize your own personal and professional values, or respond to the values of others.

- As you ask yourself these questions, focus particularly on how they may influence your future professional development. What do the answers tell you about the knowledge, skills and character which you will need to consider in order to develop?

These 'prompt questions' highlight that the reflective process requires the nurse to return to or recollect an event in order to explore and unpack behaviour, beliefs, feelings and values. It is important to recognize 'obstructing' feelings, or those aspects of recollection which are challenging or awkward. The nurse in the above example who was caring for Iain may come to consider whether she did really believe that Iain was 'stuck' with the belief that opiates were the only solution to control his pain. Instead she may consider whether she had tried to understand and respond to his own values; whether there was 'evidence' and 'knowledge' which could have helped her to understand his difficulty; or whether she had the confidence, self-belief and integrity to be the practitioner she wanted to be.

To change her future practice this nurse will first need to identify what made things difficult for her. Values-based practice involves honesty and self-awareness, and without this understanding we miss the real opportunity to learn about ourselves. Increasing our self-awareness and ability to be self-critical of our values will allow us to meet service users as people and be able to respect and listen to their views.

Summary

For centuries society has stigmatized, feared, punished and marginalized people with mental illness. We recognize today that it is a fundamental truth about mental illness that it happens to ordinary people, yet this fact may often be ignored by the media which feeds upon our prejudice and ignorance of 'others' by sensationalizing the relatively few cases where mentally ill people are a danger to the public. An emphasis on risk assessment helps to construct a public perception which exaggerates the dangerousness of those presenting with mental illness, constructs people with mental illness as different from and 'other' to ourselves, and further marginalizes and excludes people with mental illness from full participation in society.

Since the mid-1980s the involvement of service users in care has been a major political issue within health care (Thornicroft and Tansella 2005). In 2001, the DH produced a series of papers entitled *Shifting the Balance of Power*, which had the aim of empowering local communities and service users in order to ensure a health service which not only responds to individual preferences, but also is more efficient in its use of resources. Despite these policy initiatives service users still continue to feel that they are not listened to, and the fundamental observation that there should be 'no decisions about me, without me' remains an aspiration rather than reality (DH 2010b). While there is a general rhetorical commitment to service user participation, there is, however, little evidence of a widespread change of philosophy and commitment among professionals in reality (Lathlean *et al.* 2006).

The application of a values-based approach to care demonstrates a willingness to reject the 'otherness' of mental illness. A values-based philosophy of care brings with it the integrity and commitment to professional values that are the foundation for a mental health nursing practice that is truly responsive to the values of others. Adopting this approach enables us to validate the unique values and qualities of the people we care for, even when in the case of service - users such as Iain the difficulties abound and persist.

References

Beauchamp TL, Childress JF (2001) *Principles of Biomedical Ethics*, 5th edn. Oxford: Oxford University Press.

Burnard P (2002) *Learning Human Skills: An Experiential and Reflective Guide for Nurses and Health Care Professionals*, 4th edn. Oxford: Butterworth Heinemann.

Burns S, Bulman C (2000) *Reflective Practice in Nursing: The Growth of the Professional Practitioner.* Oxford: Blackwell.

Chambliss DF (1996) *Beyond Caring: Hospitals, Nurses, and the Social Organization of Ethics.* Chicago, IL: University of Chicago.

DH (2001) *Shifting the Balance of Power within the NHS.* London: The Stationery Office.

DH (2010a) *The NHS Constitution for England.* London: Department of Health.

DH (2010b) *Equity and Excellence: Liberating the NHS.* London: Department of Health.

Fulford KWM (2004) Ten principles of values based medicine, in Radden J (ed.) *The Philosophy of Psychiatry: A Companion.* New York, NY: Oxford University Press, pp. 206–34.

Fulford KWM (2011) The value of evidence and evidence of values: bringing together values-based and evidence-based practice in policy and service development in mental health. *Journal of Evaluation in Clinical Practice* 17, 976–87.

Fulford KWM, Peile E, Carroll H (2012) *Essential Values-Based Practice: Linking Science with People.* Cambridge: Cambridge University Press.

Johns C, Freshwater D (eds) (1998) *Transforming Nursing Through Reflective Practice.* Oxford: Blackwell.

Lathlean J, Burgess A, Coldham T, Gibson C, Herbert L, Levett-Jones T, Simons L, Tee S (2006) Experiences of service user and carer participation in healthcare education. *Nurse Education in Practice* **6**(6), 424–9. Online: www.sciencedirect.com/science/article/pii/S1471595306001168/accessed (6 October 2011).

MacIntyre A (1985) *After Virtue: A Study in Moral Theory*, 2nd edn. London: Duckworth.

Mohr W, Deatrick J, Richmond T, Mahon M (2001) A reflection on values in turbulent times. *Nursing Outlook* **49**(1), 30–6.

Nightingale F (1860) *Notes on Nursing: What it is, and What it is Not*, 1st American edn. New York: D. Appleton and Company.

NMC (2010) *Standards for Pre-Registration for Nursing Education*. London: Nursing Midwifery Council.

Sackett DL, Rosenburg WMC, Muir Gray JA, Haynes R, Richardson WS (1996) Evidence-based medicine: what it is and what it isn't. *British Medical Journal* **312**, 71–2.

Sackett DL, Straus SE, Richardson WS, Rosenberg W, Haynes RB (2000) *Evidence-Based Medicine: How to Practice and Teach EBM*, 2nd edn. Edinburgh: Churchill Livingstone.

Sellman D (2011) Professional values and nursing. *Medicine, Health Care and Philosophy* **14**(2), 203–8.

Thornicroft G, Tansella M (2005) Growing recognition of the importance of service user involvement in mental health service planning and evaluation. *Epidemiologia e Psichiatria Sociale* **14**(1), 1–3.

Tschudin V (2003) *Ethics in Nursing: The Caring Relationship*. Edinburgh: Butterworth-Heinemann.

University of Warwick (2010) *Values Based Practice*. Online: http://www.go.warwick.ac.uk/values-based practice (accessed 6 October 2011).

Woodbridge K, Fulford KWM (2004) *Whose Values? A Workbook for Values-Based Practice in Mental Health Care*. London: Sainsbury Centre for Mental Health.

Karen Ainsbury

Working in groups

Learning outcomes

- Understand group dynamics

- Understand the history and theory of group dynamics and group work

- Increase understanding of your own role in groups and how this can help you to understand what is happening to you in the groups that you run and their impact on you as the group leader

This chapter is split into six sections, starting with some background and history into how and why we use groups and their value. Section 2 will outline the benefits that can be gained in whatever type of group you run. The success of a group lies to a great extent in careful thinking and work in setting it up, as shown in Section 3. Sections 4–6 deal with the dynamics that can crop up throughout the lifestages of a group – beginning, middle and end. While this chapter is designed to help you spot, understand and work constructively with and in groups, it is important to remember that groups are complex and challenging and, as Nietzsche said: 'Madness is something rare in individuals – but in groups, parties, peoples, ages, it is the rule' (1886, cited in Van Der Kleij 1985, p. 102).

Therefore self-reflexive practice, as suggested in Chapter 2, plus supervision is important to help you understand the dynamics and begin to manage these challenges.

Section 1: why bring people together to work in groups?

Being a respected and effective member of the group, being accepted, being able to share, to participate, belong to the basic constructive experiences in human life. No health is conceivable without this.

(Foulkes and Anthony 1965, p. 27)

Groups are more than useful ways to impart information to more than one person at a time, they are fundamental to our sense of ourselves as human beings and key to our mental health and wellbeing – our survival in every sense. Groups are a recognized part of human evolution from clans to tribes to families. Throughout history it has been important for people to come together to hunt, gather and care for each other. Although we live in times that are described as individualist (Giddens 1992), groups remain fundamental to emotional life and we humans continue to spend most of our lives in groups – at home, at work and socially.

But groups are not just part of our social history, they are part of our neurobiological history as well. Originally, traditional neuroscience treated the nervous system as an isolated entity. Now, social neuroscience recognizes the considerable impact that social structures have on the mind and body. It shows that the brain is a single, pivotal component of an undeniably social species, and sees the brain as a social organ, whose physiological and neurological reactions are directly and profoundly shaped by social interaction (Cacioppo *et al.* 2005).

So, there is not just strength in numbers, there is also comfort, creativity and meaning to be gained by being part of a group. Neuroscience confirms what those in psychology and psychotherapy have believed from their experiences in groups – the more we engage with the people and world around us, the more our brains adapt to cope and the more we grow as individuals. How we are seen and see ourselves in groups is how we form our identity – the group situation has been likened to a hall of mirrors (Foulkes and Anthony 1965, p. 150) from whose reflections we form our self-image.

Therefore, groups can offer not only a chance for learning and intellectual development, but can also serve as an important forum for improving wellbeing and reshaping our sense of self.

The history of group work

Group work is now widely practised in mental health fields but it was not always the case. Most group work historians begin with the work of Pratt, an American chest physician, who brought together a group of patients with tuberculosis with the aim of educating them about their illness. His primary motive was to save time but he noticed that the 'fine spirit of camaraderie' (1907, p. 755), raised group members' morale and had more impact than his educational talk. As a result, he cut his talk to a couple of minutes and went on to investigate the phenomenon he had stumbled upon. He is now recognized as the father of the repressive–inspirational approach, which forms the basis for groups such as Alcoholics Anonymous (Corsini 1955).

Over the next 20 years, several others reported on the educational uses of group techniques. American psychiatrist Cody Marsh (1933) felt that the stigma of the psychiatric hospital impacted on people's ability to recover and set up classes where people could enrol as students to learn about and take responsibility for their treatment.

However, American psychoanalyst Trigent Burrow (1927) moved to a group format owing to concerns over the power dynamic of the one-to-one situation. He felt it was more egalitarian to explore the reactions of all people to each other and set up communal residences with co-workers to explore the inter-personal dynamics of groups. He is generally thought of as the forerunner of Esalen encounter-type groups, which are linked with humanistic psychology.

Freud's interest in groups was marginal. In 1922 he wrote *Group Psychology and the Analysis of the Ego*, but he was mainly concerned with the mass group phenomena found in large institutional groups such as the Church and the Army. In 1942, psycho-educationalist and psychoanalyst Fritz Redl published 'Group emotion and leadership' in *Psychiatry*, based on his observations of groups of children in holiday camps. His research showed that the activity and personality of the leader produced different group phenomena. Redl drew profiles of 'central persons' or stereotypes such as:

- *The elderly teacher*. If he is admired and loved by his pupils, he tends to have a class which is hard-working and obedient.

- *The younger teacher*. He is admired but feels more accessible because of his age and attitudes. This produces a group which is freer from disapproval.

- *The tyrannical teacher*. His class submits passively but sullenly. His group members show little friendship to each other and can turn on individuals in the style of their teacher. If, however, someone in this group rebels successfully, they can become the group hero.

At the same time, sociologists and psychologists were also investigating group processes. The experiments by Elton Mayo (1949, cited in Nichol 2000) at the Hawthorn plant in Chicago showed, among other things, that work is a group activity and that teamwork allows people to form strong working relationships and increases trust. It also found that workers are motivated by recognition, security and a sense of belonging – important aspects for all group workers to bear in mind.

These experiments began to filter into psychotherapy and mental health work with Schilder (1939, cited in Behr and Hearst 2005, p. 16), Wender (1936, cited in Behr and Hearst 2005, p. 15), Slavson (1943) and Wolf and Schwartz (1962) in the USA; Moreno (1934, cited in Foulkes 1948, p. 15) and Lewin (1947), first in Germany then in the USA; and Foulkes (1948) and Bierer (cited in Foulkes 1948, p. 18) in England working with group processes.

Although German gestalt psychologist Kurt Lewin moved to America in the 1930s, his experiences of pre-war Nazi Germany influenced his research into how social attitudes were formed and could be influenced. Like Redl he also studied the effects of leadership on groups, such as *laissez-faire*, democratic and authoritarian styles. His work led to the T-group movement (small unstructured groups used for training managers in group dynamics and leadership). However, it was large numbers of returning soldiers suffering from the psychological effects of the Second World War that propelled the work forward in Britain. Most of the people who were to shape post-war group work – Bion (1961), Main (1989), Bridger (1946, cited in Foulkes 1948, p. 17), Rickman (1943, see Bion and Rickmann (1943) below) and Foulkes (1948) – worked at Northfield Military Hospital in Birmingham during the war.

In 1943, Bion and Rickman were posted there to deal with the 'unruly' soldiers on the training wing (Kraupl Taylor 1958, p. 53). They attributed the unruly conditions to the authoritarian regime and began an ambitious scheme to replace the authority with groups that worked co-operatively. This encouraged a feeling of belonging and led the soldiers to assume some personal responsibility. The work brought Bion and Rickman into conflict with the commanding officer and they left after only six weeks but, according to Kraupl Taylor, they were still successful and morale improved. Their work is captured in a paper they wrote for *The Lancet* in 1943, 'Intra-group tensions in therapy', in which they summarized the characteristics of a good group:

- Group members share a common purpose
- The boundaries of the group are recognized
- The group has a capacity to absorb and lose members without fear of losing the group's character
- The group is free from the detrimental effects of exclusive internal sub-groups
- Each member is valued for their contribution to the group
- The group has a capacity to face and cope with internal conflict
- The minimum size of a group is three members.

Their place was taken by a team headed by SH Foulkes, who had started working with small therapeutic groups in Exeter, before moving to the hospital wing at Northfield. He writes extensively on the 'Northfield Experiment' in his book *An Introduction to Group Analytic Psychotherapy* (1948). He and his colleagues set about building on the work begun earlier by Bion and Rickmann and set up various groups transforming the hospital into the first therapeutic community.

Bion returned to the Tavistock Clinic, London, where he wrote *Experiences in Groups and Other Papers* (1961), which includes the *Lancet* paper, before moving away from group work, while Foulkes went on to establish the Institute of Group Analysis. Following his experiences at Northfield, Main (1946) extended the therapeutic community principles at the Cassel Hospital and later wrote his famous paper 'The ailment' (Main 1957), which discusses how staff teams can split and divide in response to working with people with particular psychopathology. Maxwell Jones (1952, cited in Behr and Hearst 2005, p. 25) worked with those suffering from psychosis through an integrated system of psycho-drama and community meetings at the Social Rehabilitation Unit at Belmont Hospital (Jones 1952).

What constitutes a group?

A group is more than a collection of individuals. For example, musicians playing their instruments in the same room do not make an orchestra. It needs someone to gather some of them together and give out sheet music before they can begin to play together and form a cohesive group.

As stated in the early work of Bion, in order to become a group the individuals need a common purpose. This begins to give the group a frame which is added to and strengthened by a regular meeting day or days; a regular meeting time; and a physical space to meet in. These draw important boundaries around the group. These boundaries separate group members from non-group members – those chosen for the orchestra are 'in' the group, those not given the music or invited to rehearsals are not in the group. This is important because a group needs this differentiation and focus in order to develop cohesion. The boundary also acts as an invisible psychic skin around the group that can provide containment and create a safe space in which to explore and work. Setting and monitoring the boundaries are important as disruptions – changes to time, place etc., people leaving, walking out or others intruding on the group – can upset the equilibrium of the group and its ability to attend to its task.

A group also needs a leader or co-leader/facilitator to establish these boundaries as part of what group analysts refer to as dynamic administration.

- *Administration*: because it involves you deciding what the group will be about and who it will be for. You may also find an appropriate space and set out the room for the group – ensuring enough space, seating and necessary materials such as flip charts, pens etc.

- *Dynamic*: because it requires you to actively think about the group, bringing it to life in your mind before bringing it into being in reality. The more you are able to take an active part in this the better because how you manage the administration and people's responses to it will also have dynamic implications (see Sections 4 and 5).

Section 2: benefits of working in groups

Groups offer multiple relationships to assist the individual in growth and problem-solving. The benefits of working in groups is probably best summed up by Yalom (2005), who identifies 11 'curative factors' that are the 'primary agents of change' in therapeutic groups and were derived from a series of therapy variables correlated with patient outcome. Yalom is popular on both sides of the Atlantic and his principles apply to all modalities of groups. These factors are briefly described below.

Instillation of hope

Although people come to groups to decrease their suffering and improve their lives, they are all at different stages and have different coping abilities, which can give hope and inspiration to others.

> **Case Study 4.1**
>
> Paul was in despair when he first came to the group for depression, but over time he has begun to settle and feel better. Seeing him improve has been inspirational for Elizabeth, who has felt similar to Paul at times. When John joins the group it is hard for him to believe the group leader, who he sees as not suffering in the same way, but when he hears from Paul it makes sense and gives him hope.

Universality

Many who enter groups run by mental health professionals have had difficulty sustaining inter-personal relationships, and may feel unlikable and unlovable so it is not surprising that they feel isolated or the odd one out, especially at the beginning of a group.

> **Case Study 4.1**
>
> *Continued*
>
> *Elizabeth:* There's no point me coming here. No- one ever listens to me.
>
> *Group facilitator:* That sounds very lonely Elizabeth. I wonder if anyone else recognizes that kind of feeling?
>
> *Sinead:* My family never took any notice of me so I just used to shut myself up in my room.
>
> *Ahmed:* My mother was always nagging me to come out of my room but she wasn't really interested in what I was going through.
>
> *Elizabeth:* Really, you too? I always think other people's families are more sorted than mine.

For many people, it may be the first time they feel understood and similar to others. Enormous relief often accompanies the recognition that they are not alone; this is a special benefit of group work.

Information giving

An essential component of many groups is increasing members' knowledge and understanding of a common problem. Explicit instruction about the nature of their shared illness, such as depression, panic disorders or bulimia, is often a key part of group work. Knowledge can also lead to self-management and build self-esteem.

> **Case Study 4.1**
>
> *Continued*
>
> *Elizabeth:* When I came here I just thought, 'I'm depressed, that's it!' But listening to the others and talking about our experiences and coping strategies has helped me see things in more detail. Now I can use my mood diary to spot when I am heading for a downer and do something to help myself.

Altruism

Groups offer members a unique opportunity – the chance to help others. This is important because people with mental health issues can feel as if they have little to offer others. Helping others is a powerful therapeutic tool that greatly enhances members' sense of self-worth.

Corrective recapitulation of the primary family

If people have had troubled family experiences a group can offer a chance to understand and work through troubling dynamics. Like a family, a small group of up to eight people has a leader (or co-leaders), an authority figure who can evoke feelings similar to those felt toward parents. Other group members substitute for siblings, vying for attention and affection from the leader/parent, and forming subgroups and coalitions with other members. This recasting of the family of origin gives members a chance to see, understand and work through difficult inter-personal relationships.

> **Case Study 4.1**
>
> *Continued*
>
> Angel realized that whenever she thought people were going to disagree in the group sessions she became uncomfortable and tried to make everything calm. Over time, with feedback from the facilitator and other group members, she worked out that this had been her role between her warring parents. Learning this meant she could start to practise considering her own feelings, which had previously had to be put on one side. The first time she was able to be annoyed and assertive in the group, everyone was pleased because it felt like a breakthrough.

Improved social skills

Some groups place emphasis on improving social skills; for example, with adolescents preparing to leave a psychiatric hospital, or among bereaved or divorced members seeking to date again. Group members offer feedback to one another about the appropriateness of others' behaviour. While this may be painful, the directness and honesty with which it is offered can provide much-needed behavioural correction and thus improve relationships both within and outside the group.

Making good use of personal feedback in a group is helpful but it can take time to build enough trust to be able to tell each other openly and honestly how they think and feel about what people say and do.

Case Study 4.1

Continued

Paul admitted that he was tempted to switch off when Ahmed spoke. He was embarrassed to say so but felt it was important because he liked Ahmed and wondered what it was that was causing his reaction. With the help of the other group members Paul learned that he tended to switch off when other men were speaking. Ahmed also learned that his tendency to talk without allowing spaces for people to join in left him isolated.

Imitative behaviour

As a group leader it is helpful to be aware of your own behaviour, as group members will often look to you to model helpful behaviours. For example, if you actively listen, give non-judgemental feedback and offer support, members can pick up these behaviours and try them for themselves.

Inter-personal learning

Human beings are social animals, born ready to connect. Our lives are characterized by intense and persistent relationships, and much of our self-esteem is developed via feedback and reflection from important others. Yet we all develop distortions in the way we see others, and these distortions can damage even our most important relationships. Therapy groups provide an opportunity for members to improve their ability to relate to others and live far more satisfying lives because of it.

Group cohesiveness

Belonging, acceptance and approval are among the most important and universal of human needs. Fitting in with our peers as children and adolescents, joining clubs as young adults, and joining a church or other social group as adults all fulfil these basic human needs. Many people with emotional problems, however, have not experienced success as group members. For them, group therapy may make them feel truly accepted and valued for the first time. This can be a powerful healing factor as individuals replace their feelings of isolation and separateness with a sense of belonging.

Catharsis

Catharsis is a powerful emotional experience – the release of an extreme emotion such as sorrow, fear or even hilarity – followed by a feeling of great relief. Sometimes being able to let go and experience a powerful emotion with others can lead to immediate and long-lasting change. A group environment provides ample opportunity for members to have these powerful experiences.

Case Study 4.1

Continued

As the group listened to Paul and Ahmed talk about being bullied there was a sense of tension and people began to fidget. Rosa was near to tears but suddenly burst out angrily: 'I could hit those people that did that to you!' She was shocked at her outburst but Elizabeth agreed, clenching her fists, 'They had no right to do that. I am furious when I think about what those bullies did!' It was the first time anyone in the group had managed to express anger and suddenly the whole group came to life.

Existential factors

Existential factors such as death, isolation and freedom are realities of life. Being aware of these can lead to anxiety. The trust and openness that develops among members of a longer term group can allow exploration of these fundamental issues. For example, losing people from a group can lead to discussions and exploration of feelings around loss and death. It can help members to accept and develop a resilience in the face of difficult realities.

Section 3: setting up a group

Groups take many shapes and guises. The format, frequency and membership of your group may not always be in your control. However, if you have an opportunity to have an input into this, it can be helpful where possible to think carefully about setting up your group. You cannot plan for every eventuality, but preparation is important. You would not throw seeds on unprepared ground and hope they will grow. With a group, groundwork is all important.

Questions of administration

1. *What size of group*? How many members will it have? A group can be as small as three, according to Bion (1961; see Table 4.1). What is the most people you will or can take?

Table 4.1 Impact of group size

Small group	8–12 people. This is family sized and is best if you want to encourage insight and the sharing of personal or intimate information
Median group	12–30 people. Less comfortable for sharing personal information. More reminiscent of a classroom size and is more suitable for matters of the mind than the heart. It is a good place to practise dialogue and social skills but will need to break down into smaller groups for more intimate sharing. The size can exacerbate feelings of alienation or loss of identity
Large group	30+. This is more of a representation of society at large and is likely to bring up wider issues regarding cultures. The issues around the sharing of information are increased from the median group

2. *Where will it be held*? This can affect how many people you can see, what you can do and timings. Try to pick a venue that is suitable and conveniently situated for your membership. For example, one NHS Trust held groups for people with a diagnosis of borderline personality disorder in local sports team clubs because they were easy to get to, available during the day and removed from the hospital environment.

3. *When will it be held*? Again this can have an impact on membership. The easier you make it to get to – for example matching with transport timings – the more people are likely to get there.

4. *Will you run it alone*? Is it possible to run the group single-handed? Working with a co-facilitator can free you up to pay attention to different aspects of the work, e.g. one can lead exercises while the other observes reactions and helps to take care of members who might be struggling. Working with others can help if you are managing a large group.

5. *How long can you commit to*? This is likely to be more important if you are thinking of running a group for several months or if you plan for the group to be handed on to others at a later date. A group can be quite a commitment. It is easier to change times and places when working with an individual but much harder when you have a number of people to consider. Also, even if only two or three people turn up – as can happen particularly around holiday times or the end of a group – the group still runs and needs your full commitment. Losing the leader can be a major blow to a longer term group and affect its stability (see Section 6).

6. *How long will it run? Both in number of sessions and length of sessions*? What is the ideal number of sessions for what you are trying to achieve? Also ask yourself how long you will need to get through what you hope in each session – particularly if you are mixing exercises and a bit of teaching with discussion. Remember the lessons learned by Pratt (see Section 1) and leave enough time for the discussion as this is important for the group to gel and begin to feel a sense of personal agency.

7. *How will they get to you/get in*? This might sound a little over-detailed but many is the group that has sat waiting for members to arrive only to later discover that they were stopped by receptionists, locked out or wandering round looking for the room – the

last is a particular problem in the early stages of a group or for new members joining a long-running group.

Questions around format

There are so many types, styles and sizes of groups to choose from that the task of setting one up can be quite bewildering. To help, Dorothy Stock Whitaker has devised a simple, three-dimensional grid (cited in Barnes *et al.* 1999, p. 5), which links together:

1. Who do you want to work with? (what type of condition, issue or service user?)

2. What do you hope to achieve?

   and, considering the two above

3. How can the group be set up for these people in order to achieve this?

Let us take a couple of group examples and answer these questions: Group A – Living with depression; Group B – Preparing for discharge.

Group A – Living with depression

Who do you hope to work with?

This could be a group for those with a diagnosis of chronic depression, e.g. more than five years in duration. Members could be of differing ages and backgrounds but have in common that they are socially isolated and/or unable to work.

What do you hope to achieve?

A reduction in symptoms of depression (according to whatever measure you are using) and an increase in social functioning as a result of reduced feelings of isolation, i.e. able to join social groups or return to work.

What kind of group can be set up to achieve this?

- A small group (8–10) will make this less daunting for people who find social interaction difficult and allow for corrective recapitulation of the primary family (see Table 4.1).

- The group needs to meet regularly, at a fixed time, so that it becomes a reliable space. This group will also meet weekly to help members to gel – holding on to new relationships is harder when the gaps between meetings are longer. All will help with group cohesiveness (see text).

- It will run for one and a half hours, to allow some space for exercises and teaching and plenty of time for discussion. Remember Pratt's findings that what people learn from each other promotes a sense of self-worth and feeling of being able to care for one's self.

- This group will run in the afternoon as many people with clinical depression find it hard to get up in the morning and find their mood improves as the day progresses and are therefore more likely to be motivated to attend at a later time.

continued ➤

- It will be a slow-open group, which means that the group itself will have no fixed finishing date. A minimum of five people will enable the group to start and others can join as they are referred and assessed as suitable. However, individuals will be offered a fixed period in the group of 18 months. This will give enough time to do some meaningful work but will encourage people to consider how they can move on and fit into other groups with more varied membership – whether this is social/work/education groups or maybe a support group if necessary.

- The slow-open format will mean that members will be at varying stages of development, allowing for Yalom's instillation of hope, and will also enable group members to grapple with existential factors such as new people, competition and loss.

- Firm boundaries will be needed to make the group safe enough to encourage open and honest inter-personal learning.

- The group could be used to teach the members a little about their condition and help them share their differing experiences of their illness, swap coping strategies and learn new ones. It could be used to help members use each other as mirrors in order to understand behaviours, etc. which reinforce their symptoms and limit their lifestyles – it is often easier to spot traits and habits in others than in ourselves. This will need to be sensitively handled by the facilitators so that it is encouraging rather than judgemental.

Group B – Preparing for discharge

Who is it for?

People actively preparing to leave a day hospital and some who are, at this stage, exploring the idea of discharge. Those leaving may need help managing the transition in order to sustain their improved mental health without the daily support of the hospital. Others might attend to begin to think about themselves as potential leavers.

What do you hope to achieve?

It can be quite a shock to the system to go from daily support and purpose to going it alone or returning sometimes to family life or other situations that might test new coping skills or tentative steps of recovery. This group will help people to explore the issues they might face such as potential loneliness; lack of confidence; a rise in anxiety; and how to access other support if necessary. It will provide a forum for people to discuss leaving and possible concerns. It will also provide skill-building exercises and useful information.

What kind of group can be set up to achieve this?

- This will be fixed term group and will run weekly for eight, two-hour sessions. It will have up to 12 members and will be run by day hospital staff members and a colleague from the community mental health team – linking the two worlds the group intends to bridge. Two facilitators means the group can be split easily into two smaller groups for some of the exercises and more in-depth discussion. There will be refreshments and a generally social feeling to the group.

- The group will use a broadly cognitive behavioural framework, encouraging members to examine their thoughts and how this affects feelings, how behaviours affect mood and the link to physiological responses. It will look at issues such as: goal-setting; assertiveness; anxiety management; and alternative social groups and activities.
- The group will also have an outing on week seven, to encourage members to take part in social activities outside the day centre.
- The ending of the group will be used to mirror the loss of leaving the hospital and help members express, understand and normalize their feelings around loss.
- Useful feedback and ideas from members will be considered and taken up to enhance the discharge process where possible.

Questions for prospective members

The clearer you are about what the group is for, the easier it will be for you to choose people who will benefit. It will also be easier for people to imagine themselves as part of the group. However, it is important to think beyond gathering people for a group and to think about how you can help them stay in the group.

Communication is key: you might have people in mind for your group, but they might not agree. The main contraindication for group membership is not wanting to do it. If at all possible, it is helpful to see people individually first to assess their suitability for your group and to allow them to explore the idea of the group. If you cannot meet them individually, these issues could be tackled in a pre-group session, or even, if need be, the first group session.

Tell them about the group and why you are inviting them to join – being chosen can feel good, but that glow can soon wear off in a group of strangers when you are anxious. These meetings are particularly important if colleagues have referred people to your group and you do not know them. Useful issues for you and prospective group members to explore are:

- *Where will it be held*? Holding initial meetings in the group venue can help prospective members begin to get a feel for the group and imagine how it might be to take part. Knowledge of the venue – the room, layout, where the toilets are – will help to ease anxiety at the first meeting.

- *How do they imagine others will be*? We all imagine, it is human nature, and this can allow fears to come up and be discussed. Along with this, you might wonder together what kind of things they are expecting to happen. This will give you a chance to see if what you are hoping to offer matches their expectations. It also gives you a chance to explore things that might not appear on a neat planning sheet. For example, someone might fear another person bursting into tears or they might have bladder control problems and need to know how their leaving the room might be handled. These kinds of things can torment people and lead them to not show up or drop out of groups for fear of shame. Simple enquiries such as 'What kind of thing would make you uncomfortable in this group?' or 'How might you react and what can we think of together to help you or stop you walking out?' can help to bring the group alive and can take the shock or sting out of events if and when they do happen. You also need to consider:

- How do you think you will be in the group? (talk all the time; say nothing, etc.).
- How are you in other groups?
- What kind of groups have they been in? (this can include school classes, family gatherings, as well as social groups etc.).
- How did they experience those groups? What made it good, difficult, boring, frightening etc.?
- Did they stay? How did it end?

Looking for patterns at this stage (see Case Study 4.2) will help you gain an idea of the person as a group member and help them to make a smoother transition into a group.

Case Study 4.2

Simon said he was keen to be in the group and Della was tempted to stop the preparation meeting there but she asked him what other groups he belonged to or had belonged to in the past? Simon said he had tried a few night classes but didn't really get on with them. They always seemed like a good idea but he usually got bored. Della realized that Simon might be keen to start her group like the night classes but might not stay the course. By exploring what led him to drop out of classes they found that Simon would often fall behind with the work and then feel it was pointless staying. They were then able to work out how they would spot when this might be happening in the new group and how they would tackle it to help him see the course through this time. Della realized that this would not only help Simon to stay and increase what he learned, it had the potential to give him a new experience of learning and of himself and would be important for his self-development.

Questions for you

Even if you are the person running the group, you are still *part* of the group and it can be equally useful to ask yourself some of the questions you ask prospective group members. How you feel in groups and how you run them will affect the responses from group members (see Section 1).

> **Reflective Exercise 4.1**
>
> **What sort of groups do you like?**
> Think about your positive and negative experiences in groups.
>
> - What was it that made them positive or negative?
> - Was it size, membership, leadership, task, content, context?
> - Perhaps it was a combination of these or something else?
> - How do all these factors impact on how you experience groups and how you expect groups to be?

Avoiding isolates

Isolation is linked to exclusion and can feel threatening and anxiety provoking, it is important to avoid, where possible, people who will stand out as obviously different from the group you are putting together.

> **Case Study 4.3**
>
> - Rosie is a 42-year-old mother of three who has never worked.
> - Sharon is a 47-year-old woman who is childless and works.
> - Martin is a 39-year-old father of two who is unemployed. His wife works.
>
> Although these people are different they have obvious links around work and they are similar ages. It might be more difficult for Sharon if she is the only person in the group who has no children. It would mark Martin apart if he was the only man. Overt religious or political views can also separate individuals from the crowd. People with depression, anxiety and other mental health issues can often feel the 'odd one out'. If they arrive at a group in which they are isolated for some reason, the group experience can be extremely undermining. For your members' comfort and for group cohesion to stand a good chance it is helpful to pick people who have links.

While it is not impossible to work with these situations, it can become harder for people to form important associations and feel connected to others. Thus it can lead to scapegoating and drop-outs.

Section 4: group dynamics

Some groups allow more space for understanding and reflecting on the inter-personal dynamics between members – a personal development group, or reflective practice group. Others allow this aspect to drift into the background and focus more on task, e.g.

managing stress, coping with panic attacks. Whatever modality or format your group takes, *it will have group dynamics*, as the teams at Northfield discovered (see Section 1), and understanding a little about these dynamics will help to you set up and run more successful groups. The added benefit of considering the group's dynamics is that it helps to make the things you are working on in the group live and relational rather than just theoretical.

Those dynamics also involve you and anyone who runs the group with you. At the outset, you will have the role of picking members and deciding on the focus of the work as well as setting the time, day and location of the group. This is a powerful position and will have an impact on the dynamics. When it is running, you are part of the group, albeit in a different role. An understanding of groups and their impact on you will also serve to strengthen your ability to help the group run effectively.

Group dynamics start before the group

Jerome Bruner (1990) said: 'When we enter human life, it is as if we walk on stage into a play whose enactment is already in progress – a play whose somewhat open plot determines what part we may play and toward what denouements we may be heading' (p. 34). Bruner was talking about birth into our families – our entry into the first group in life. What he was suggesting is that life is not a blank piece of paper, but is already scripted to some extent according to existing family dynamics. This might include your position in the family, your gender and how you are thought about in the family; and whether it is a large family, a wealthy one, and so on.

Add to the above wider social and cultural factors, such as religion, social status, ethnic origin, religion, country of birth, and we have what is referred to as our foundation matrix (Foulkes 1975). Our foundation matrix is important because it affects the way individuals behave in groups and expect to be received and understood by others. It impacts on the way we communicate both explicitly through speech and body language, gestures and actions and unconsciously in our approach to others, our values and our prejudices.

> These primary levels [of communication – inflexions of voice; manner of speaking; looking; expressions; gestures; actions; emotional reactions] correspond to the foundation matrix, based on the biological properties of the species, but also on the culturally firmly embedded values and reactions. These have been developed and transmitted, especially in the nuclear family, in the social network, class, etc. and have been maintained or modified by the intimate plexus in which the person now moves.
>
> (Foulkes 1975, p. 131, original emphasis)

Therefore, the foundation matrix of your group members is likely to have an impact on your group and the way it functions – how people speak to each other, or stay silent, who feels they can speak to whom. You will pick some of this up at your introductory meetings, if you have been able to have them.

Case Study 4.4

The Living with Depression group was meant to be discussing situations where members wanted to be more assertive and think about their rights, but it had slipped into what Della thought of as 'coffee morning chat'. She found herself becoming irritated and started coming up with ideas for them as she felt they would run out of time.

When she discussed it with her supervisor, he asked if she seemed to be the only one who seemed to get cross. Della realized that was so. The supervisor pointed out that Della had grown up with people taking her seriously and being able to stand up for her rights. Della realized that she was behaving according to her script and the group members were acting according to theirs.

The following week she went back to the group and put her thoughts into words, rather than acting on them. She said that she was tempted to come up with ideas for them and instead gave more time to explore what they thought would happen to their ideas *if* they had them. Most group members then began to share ideas but added that they would not happen or had failed in the past (their fixed script). She then asked them to imagine a story in which a character played them and did things differently – this freed people up to begin to rewrite their scripts.

The conductor's script

You may be the group 'leader', the 'facilitator' or the 'convenor'. Group analysts tend to favour the term 'conductor', first coined by social theorist TW Adorno (1950, cited in Behr and Hearst 2005, p. 7) and adopted by Foulkes (1975), who liked the idea of the fluctuating authority between the conductor and the orchestra.

The conductor not only needs to lead practice and know music but also needs to actively listen to help the musicians work together to make music. Conductors and orchestras often bring their own interpretations to a piece of music depending on their skills, composition and background – the music they have grown up with and studied. The conductor brings people in at the appropriate moments and also needs to develop a sensitive ear to discordant notes, people playing different tunes, refrains that keep appearing, etc. – these make up the dynamics of the group. An ear for these and an open exploration of them, rather than dismissal, can lead to creativity.

To help you develop your 'ear' it helps to know your natural role in groups. As you can see in Case Study 4.4, Della was using herself and her own reactions to tune into the unconscious rhythms of the group. This is another aspect to the therapeutic use of self discussed in Chapter 2. The more familiar you are with your own feelings about groups and in groups, the more comfortable you will be running a group and tackling any difficulties that may arise.

Reflective Exercise 4.2

Uncovering your group script

Take a moment to think about some of the groups you have taken part in during your life and that you are influenced by: family (and your position in it); society; social/socio-economic group; sex and sexuality; location (town/country, etc.); schools/workplaces; religion. You are likely to come up with many more.

How did they affect your 'play setting' or 'script'? What other factors played their part? Divorce, loss, adoption, changing countries? Other life events?

Reflective Exercise 4.3

What part or parts do you play in groups?
- What sort of group member are you?
- What part do you play?
- Do you behave differently in different groups or do you have a fairly consistent pattern?

Some group roles are: joker; peace-maker; rescuer; observer; rebel; competitor; outsider; conductor; carer; teacher; go-between; victim; martyr (you may come up with others).

Early dynamics and its effects

Going into a new group can be nerve-wracking for anyone. People wonder if they will fit in or be judged. Through your initial interviews you might know what people have in common and the potential for connections but, until these come to the surface, the group is just 'a collection of individuals who have no relationship with each other, other than the common task of forming the group' (Nitsun 1989, p. 250). Nitsun linked the early stages of a long-term therapeutic group to the early development of the infant – the first 12 weeks of the group to the first three months of infancy. In both instances, he says, the major task is integration and both need a 'good enough' carer who is attentive and can manage this anxiety.

This can be useful to bear in mind when bringing together any group of people who have not met before and whom you hope will come, in a short time, to share their private thoughts, hopes and fears. Although people come to groups in the hope of finding support, relief from symptoms and a sense of togetherness, trust takes time to develop and there can be fear of attack and hostility. As the conductor, rather like the lightning conductor which channels the electricity, you might also be able to feel something of the anxiety. While your group members may lapse into silence or talk endlessly to cover their fears, it will be your role to model care and concern and illustrate how the group will work.

Case Study 4.4

Continued

Only four people had arrived by the time Della was due to start her new group. She welcomed those present and said that she was expecting two more members (indicating the two empty chairs waiting for them) as they had not contacted her to say they could not make the group. But she would be starting on time and the others could join in as they arrived: *this reiterated the time boundaries that the group would start and finish on time and also let members know that their role was to let her know in advance if they could not make a session.*

After people had told each other their names, they fell silent and Della wondered if it had something to do with the missing people. She felt anxious to press on but, as part of the group task was to learn how to put feelings into words and be more assertive, she decided to model staying with concerns and exploring them.

Della noticed that people were finding it rather hard to get started and wondered why that might be? John said he felt it was better to wait for the others to arrive. A couple of others agreed, while Sinead said she would rather get on but it didn't matter. Della acknowledged the differing views and wondered how the members present might feel if they had been delayed. They were just talking about how they might like people to welcome them, when the door opened a crack. Della smilingly waved the newcomer in.

It can be tricky to strike a balance like Della in Case Study 4.4. She acknowledged all the views and noticed that Sinead was in danger of being a lone voice. Rather than singling her out, Della helped the group to move on while considering the missing people: this conductor is taking an active and inclusive role; she is open to difference and containing.

Section 5: mid-group dynamics

Some group workers prefer to think of working with individuals in a group setting, while others focus on the group task and look at the group 'as a whole' in relation to the task (Bion 1961). Whichever you choose to focus on, the other will always be present and it is possible to work in a way which holds both in mind. Like modern-day social neuroscientists, Foulkes (1948) saw people as individuals impacted by their social contexts and suggested that we look at groups as the form of a 'figure and ground gestalt' – sometimes when we look we see the individual set against the backdrop of the group; look again and we see the group dynamics impacting on individuals.

> At the centre of all our thinking about communication in groups is the concept of the group network or group matrix … The group is a matrix of interpersonal relationships, and the events which occur in it are interpersonal phenomena. These relationships and these events exist literally in between two or more people; they do not occur in one person or in another, but can only come into existence through the interaction of two or more people.

> (Foulkes and Anthony 1965, p. 258)

What this means is that, while it is important to pay attention to the thoughts, feelings, words and actions of the individual, it can also be helpful to stop and consider if the individual is expressing something that the group may be feeling or struggling with. This concept underpins other group phenomena such as scapegoating (see Section 5). It also suggests that although group members begin their group experience governed mainly by their foundation matrix, which draws on their experiences of past groups, members go on to develop a 'dynamic matrix', which grows and develops between existing group members.

> All [the foundation matrix] … is now temporarily replaced by the artificially created, strange but potentially very intimate group network... This dynamic matrix is in fact the theatre of operation of ongoing change.

> (Foulkes 1975, p. 132, original emphasis)

Stacey (2003) refers to this 'theatre of change' as the 'living present' because it provides a living, breathing, current opportunity for people to relate differently to each other in the present moment. It is more powerful than theory or role play because it harnesses the real relationships in the group (see Case Study 4.5).

Stopping drop-outs

If arriving late becomes a habit rather than the occasional one-off, it can be useful in your group to explore what is behind it, as it could be a precursor to dropping out. Remember to model friendly curiosity rather than judgement. Although you are more likely to lose people at the beginning when people have not formed attachments to each other, changes in group format throughout the life of the group can cause these early anxieties to re-emerge because a *changed* group is, in effect, a *new* group to some degree.

A member choosing to leave a group, either because they are ready to leave or for other reasons – ill health, change of home circumstances, etc. – can cause a ripple effect and other members suddenly feel it is time for them to leave. Making space to explore the impact on the group and its members can make the ending a useful experience for all.

Case Study 4.4

Continued

James was leaving Della's group. He felt ready to leave and discussions in the group showed that most people agreed. In the few weeks before his ending, Ann said that she felt it was probably time for her to go too. Raj started arriving late, or not showing, which was unusual. Bearing the idea of figure and ground in mind, Della noticed the individual behaviours but also wondered if this might be part of a bigger reaction in the group to James, one of the founder members, leaving.

Further enquiry helped Della and the members to understand that their behaviour was linked to James's leaving. Ann realized she had started at the same time as James and felt she should be ready to go at the same time, without acknowledging how things really felt for her. Raj felt sad and angry at James for leaving. He was behaving according to his family script and avoiding the ending by turning up late. The group was then able to discuss their different attitudes to leaving, how it affected their behaviour and how it impacted on their lives – such as leaving them isolated, or with physical symptoms such as a tight chest and headaches because they were carrying thoughts and feelings around that were not expressed.

James was tempted to stay when he listened to Ann and Raj, but the group helped him to see that leaving was right for him and that he would not be forgotten. For James it was the first time he felt he would be missed but did not have to feel guilty.

Changes in leadership

Any comings and goings, particularly in a longer term group, can destabilize the dynamics. If you as group leader are off for any reason – sickness, holiday, a course – your absence can evoke unconscious feelings around attachment and separation.

Remember that you have been responsible for bringing this group into being and setting the boundaries which form its psychic skin. Your sudden absence can undermine feelings of security and perhaps even trigger unconscious feelings of disregard or abandonment. That does not mean you should never take a break, but it does require you to model how you hope others might behave by giving due notice, where possible, and allowing space for people to consider and express their reactions to your absence.

Consider how you would feel if you turned up at your fitness class, reading group or a social gathering to find the person you were familiar with and expected to be running things had been replaced by a stranger. Would you feel put out? Hostile? Disengaged?

Disclosure

In groups it is likely that, at some point, members might share painful and distressing thoughts and experiences with each other – perhaps fears around leaving the day hospital or stories about crises that brought them to hospital. This can deepen relationships, bring healing and development (see Section 3). However, timing is important, as members can also feel exposed, hurt or ashamed. Groups need time to build up their resources to manage such disclosures. Detailed revelations made before the group is cohesive can lead to the member dropping out or others leaving if they feel the disclosure puts the pressure on to 'tell all'. Be cautious of prompting people to go into too much personal detail or depth in the first few sessions.

Another element of disclosure that can catch us unaware is the 'door handle comment' – when someone drops a bombshell just before the end of the group session, e.g. to say they are leaving, or a personal trauma. The challenge is to hold it within the boundary of the group while not going over time.

It can be enough to simply acknowledge that something important has been said and it is a shame that there is not sufficient time to discuss it this time, but that it sounds important and the group would discuss it at the next meeting. This response can stop the group being paralysed, or pulled into going over its boundaries. When the boundaries change, the group changes and this will bring back anxiety.

It can also prevent something important from being lost or squeezed out of the group, which brings us to our next topic.

Scapegoating

The term comes from the ancient Hebrew tradition where the tribe cleansed themselves of their sins by loading them onto a goat which was then sent into the desert. Their sins went with it. In modern thinking we are not ridding ourselves of our sins so much as uncomfortable feelings.

Case Study 4.5

Karl noticed that Soraya had all the right answers when it came to assertiveness theory but left the room when the Hospital Discharge group broke into smaller groups to discuss how they felt about being assertive with family members and each other. To make sure it was a pattern, he paid closer attention the next time they were in small groups. Sure enough, Soraya left and the rest settled into chatting, without challenging each other. When Soraya stood to leave for a third week, Karl decided to act in the living present and said: 'I have noticed that you sometimes leave during these sessions and I am concerned that you might be missing out on something which is important for you.' Soraya stopped, then said that she couldn't stay. He noticed that she was shaking and commented on this, asking her if she would like to sit down. She did. Eventually, she told the group how she usually went to the ladies room and waited for the group to be over in case arguments broke out. Someone else in the group said they felt the same and was glad when they just chatted but it also felt disappointing. Another group member remembered Soraya saying how it was hard to speak up in families when all people did was shout. Karl said they could think about this group like a sort of family – but one that could manage differences of opinion without becoming abusive. Soraya stayed and the group members began a discussion where they expressed differing views with some force and feeling.

It seemed that no one in this small group had wanted to wear the mantle of angry or disagreeable person – Soraya least of all. It is the fact that she had least tolerance for it that led to her walking out of the room and the group unconsciously scapegoated her, as if their difficult feelings could go with her. Keeping Soraya in the room enabled the feelings to be redistributed and allowed members to express the passion and potency that were important for them to be truly assertive.

Managing conflict

Conflict is inevitable and potentially healthy, but there is a fine line between open and honest exchanges and aggression that can be destructive. It helps to keep things in proportion. Sensibilities and egos might be wounded in groups, as in real life, but it will help to have some agreed group boundaries such as no physical contact, no slamming doors and no kicking chairs.

When discussing group rules at the beginning of groups you will find that some members want rules that will restrict real engagement between people. For example, 'Talk, don't shout', 'Treat each other with respect' – these can be secret codes for no conflict. Such hard and fast rules can lead to important discussions and feelings going underground, or lead to drop-outs. After all, when people are genuinely angry they are not always quiet and respectful.

If two people become locked in abuse toward each other, it needs to be stopped by the conductor. Here, the approach taken by mentalization-based therapists can be useful – stop, rewind, explore. The facilitator stops the interaction and insists the session rewinds to a point where constructive discussion was taking place and people were able to think about each other (Bateman and Fonagy 2006).

Stop, rewind, explore

Let's go back and see what happened just then

At first you seemed to understand what was going on but then …

Let's try to trace exactly how that came about

Hang on, before we move off, let's just rewind and see if we can understand something in all this

(Bateman and Fonagy 2006, p. 133)

Section 6: endings and leavings

All life is a process of attaching and letting go and the ending of a group provides an opportunity for members to recognize and understand more about their attachment and how they manage separation and loss. Bowlby (1981, p. 7) said that the loss of a loved person is one of the most intensely painful experiences any human being can suffer. It is also painful to witness in others because we feel impotent to help.

Although the end of the group is not a death, it can still be emotionally charged, particularly in long-standing groups, as it will resonate with endings that members have experienced in their lives – separation, loss, perhaps abandonment, and of course death. Children who experience unpredictable and intermittent emotional connection can grow into adults who need constant reassurance and find any separation too painful to tolerate. Those who were constantly rejected in their attempts to connect learn to guard themselves against emotional attachment to protect themselves from the pain of possible rejection. This fear of intimacy can show itself in disengagement either physically or emotionally before the end of a group in order to avoid potential failure, disappointment and pain.

A fixed term or closed group will be aware of its ending from its beginning, as the date will be set. However, group members can make all sorts of defensive manoeuvres to avoid the difficult feelings connected with endings.

You might find they somehow book another appointment to coincide with the final session, or simply do not arrive. Once again, paying attention to the process enables group members to begin to understand their approaches to endings and attachment, which are key to their wellbeing.

Case Study 4.6

Kirsten had decided, after years of running a group, that it was time to end. She had given the members three months' notice and had encouraged them to think about the ending and what it might mean. Members talked about what they had gained and also their disappointments – what they might like to have done.

On the last day, Isabel arrived half an hour late and admitted she had gone shopping to avoid the group. Then she had thought about her granddad's funeral, which her parents had felt she was too young to go to: 'They stopped me then but I think I've been stopping myself from going to things since. This feels like giving myself something I missed out on.'

As a final exercise, think about group endings in your life and how they have affected you.

Reflective Exercise 4.4

Group endings
- What do you think you learned from your family about responding to loss or absence?
- What are your customs and practices, for example, around the death of a family member?
- Is it acceptable to grieve openly? In what way? For how long?
- Are people who have left or died talked about in the family group? If yes, how are they spoken about?
- What makes a 'good ending' for you?
- How do you think these experiences might affect the way you think about or approach endings in groups?

Conclusion

Groups are a microcosm of life and can be complex and daunting places but also extremely rewarding. They offer a chance to understand and develop life skills and improve wellbeing. If you are to make the most of the groups that you run it can help to tune into and work with the dynamics. Employing record-keeping that is meaningful as well as statistical, and having your own debriefing and support, perhaps in supervision or a peer support group, are important.

While keeping a record of attendance is essential, keeping track of other boundary issues is also important, such as: Who turns up late and when? Are absences linked to group breaks or stand-in facilitators? Do certain people sit together? Are seating patterns rigid or flexible? Do certain people dominate the talking? Who is silent and how can they be helped to find their voice? These can all flag up patterns which can help you to explore if people are engaged or on the edge of dropping out; and allow you to do your best to keep the group together and make it a rich experience.

There are so many types and styles of group that they could not possibly be covered in one chapter; however, all groups have the same potential benefits and dynamics under the surface that will affect the success of your groups. This chapter has outlined some key aspects and given examples that will help you to identify and work with the group dynamics to the benefit of all those taking part, including the conductor.

References

Barnes B, Ernst S, Hyde K (1999) *An Introduction to Groupwork – A Group-Analytic Perspective.* London: MacMillan Press.

Bateman A, Fonagy P (2006) *Mentalization-Based Treatment for Borderline Personality Disorder: A Practical Guide.* Oxford: Oxford University Press.

Behr H, Hearst L (2005) *Group Analytic Psychotherapy: A Meeting of Minds.* London: Whurr.

Bion WR (1961) *Experiences in Groups and Other Papers.* London: Tavistock Publications.

Bowlby J (1981) *Attachment and Loss, Volume III: Loss.* London: Penguin.

Bridger H (1946) *The Northfield Experiment,* in Foulkes SH (ed.) *An Introduction to Group Analytic Psychotherapy.* London: Karnac Books.

Bruner J (1990) *Acts of Meaning.* London: Harvard University Press.

Burrow T (1927) The group method of analysis. *Psychoanalytic Review* **10**, 268–80.

Cacioppo J, Visser P, Pickett C (2005) *Social Neuroscience: People Thinking about Thinking People.* Boston, MA: MIT Press.

Corsini RG (1955) Historic background of group psychotherapy: a critique. *Group Psychotherapy* **8**(3), 219–26.

Foulkes SH (1948) *An Introduction to Group Analytic Psychotherapy.* London: Karnac Books.

Foulkes SH (1975) *Group Analytic Psychotherapy Methods and Principles.* London: Karnac Books.

Foulkes SH, Anthony EJ (1965) *Group Psychotherapy, the Psychoanalytic Approach,* 2nd edn. London: Karnac Books.

Freud S (1922) *Group Psychology and the Analysis of the Ego.* New York, NY: Boni and Liveright.

Giddens A (1992) *The Transformation of Intimacy.* Oxford: Blackwell.

Jones M (1952) *Social Pychiatry. A Study of Therapeutic Communities.* London: Tavistock Publications and Routledge and Kegan.

Kraupl Taylor F (1958) A history of group and administrative therapy in Great Britain. *British Journal of Medical Psychology* **31**, 153–73.

Lewin K (1947) Frontiers in group dynamics: concept, method and reality in social science. Social equilibria and social change. *Human Relations* **1**, 5–41.

Main TF (1946) The hospital as a therapeutic institution. *Bulletin of the Menninger Clinic* **10**, 66–70.

Main TF (1957) The ailment. *British Journal of Medical Psychology* **30**, 129–45.

Main T (1989) *The Ailment and Other Psychoanalytic Essays.* London: Free Association Books.

Marsh LC (1933) An experiment in group treatment of patients at Worcester State Hospital. *Mental Hygiene* **17**, 396–416.

Moreno JL (1934) Who will survive?, in Foulkes SH (ed.) *An Introduction to Group Analytic Psychotherapy*. London: Karnac Books.

Nichol B (2000) *Bion and Foulkes at Northfield: The Early Development of Group Psychotherapy in Britain*. Business Coach Institute. Online: www.businesscoachinstitute. com/library/bion_and_foulkes_at_northfield.shtml (accessed 6 September 2011).

Nitsun M (1989) Early development: linking the individual and the group. *Group Analysis* **22**, 249–60.

Pratt JH (1907) The class method of treating consumption in the homes of the poor. *Journal of the American Medical Association* **49**, 755–9.

Redl F (1942) Group emotion and leadership. *Psychiatry: Journal for the Study of Interpersonal Processes* **5**, 573–96.

Schilder P (1939) Results and problems of group psychotherapy in severe neurosis. *Mental Hygiene* **23**, 87–98.

Slavson SR (1943) *An Introduction to Group Therapy*. Oxford: Oxford University Press.

Stacey R (2003) *Complexity and Group Processes: A Radically Social Understanding of Individuals*. Hove: Brunner-Routledge.

Van Der Kleij G (1985) The group and its matrix. *Group Analysis* **8**, 102–10.

Wender L (1936) The dynamics of group psychotherapy and its application. *Journal of Nervous and Mental Diseases* **84**, 54–60.

Wolf A, Schwartz EK (1962) *Psychoanalysis in Groups*. New York, NY: Grune and Stratton.

Yalom ID (2005) *The Theory and Practice of Group Therapy*. New York, NY: Basic Books.

Recovery: a journey of discovery

Learning outcomes

- Be able to critically reflect on what 'recovery' means to people who have faced the challenges of emotional distress, those who have used mental health services and those who continue to experience emotional and cognitive challenges

- Evaluate the significance of family and friends, their contribution to the support of people who experience mental health problems, and their double journey of recovery – for themselves and for the person they care about

- Be able to critically analyse the values and goals of a recovery-focused approach and the fundamental changes this approach could make to care planning and service configurations

Introduction

An understanding of recovery, as defined by people who themselves experience mental health problems, has the potential to transform the approaches used, interventions offered and values held by people who provide services. Such changes in services, in turn, have the potential to transform the experience of mental health problems from a devastating, catastrophic, life-destroying occurrence to a challenge that can be managed and which ultimately enriches us all; and broadens our understanding, contribution and sensitivity towards others. Note: this chapter will move from speaking about 'you' as the person who might understand what it is like to suffer from mental distress and/or a diagnosis to 'you' the trainee or practitioner who wants to help people who are in emotional distress.

A recovery-focused approach is consistent with the Nursing and Midwifery Council's (NMC) competency framework. In particular, it provides a framework within which mental health nurses can:

- Practise in a holistic, non-judgemental, caring and sensitive manner that: avoids assumptions; supports social inclusion; recognizes and respects individual choice; and acknowledges diversity. Where necessary, they must challenge inequality, discrimination and exclusion from access to care.

- Support and promote the health, wellbeing, rights and dignity of people, groups, communities and populations. These include people whose lives are affected by ill health, disability, ageing, death and dying, and understand how these activities influence public health.

- Work in partnership with service users, carers, families, groups, communities and organizations; manage risk; and promote health and wellbeing while aiming to empower choices that promote self-care and safety.

To be diagnosed with mental health problems is a catastrophic and life-changing experience. Perhaps those ordinary everyday things you have always done without thinking have become impossibly difficult. Maybe you have to cope with strange and frightening experiences that no one around you believes or understands. Possibly you do things that are out of character. But it is not simply the difficulties that led to your diagnosis that are challenging. It is all that it means to be defined as a 'mental patient' in our society with all the prejudice and stereotypes that abound and the discrimination and exclusion that result. It is not just the big things, like the risk of losing your job or friends, or college place. Even at a day-to-day level people start treating you differently. Maybe they avoid you or stop believing what you say – start 'humouring' you, or treat you like a child. The 'us' and 'them' divide continues to separate those diagnosed as 'mentally ill' from those who are not both within and outside mental health services.

It is not surprising that the whole experience of becoming a 'mental patient' leads people to lose confidence in themselves and leads to a feeling of being very alone and frightened:

- Frightened about what is happening to you
- Frightened about trusting your own judgement
- Frightened about the prospect of using mental health services
- Frightened that you will lose everything you value in life, like your friends, your work, your home, your college place, your position in the community
- Frightened that you won't be able to achieve your ambitions – do all the things you had planned to do in life like raise a family, travel, get a good job.

I lost valuable years of my life … some dreams went out of the window … but I feel stronger than ever now … and wiser. I am content … I am very into my music and performing, making tracks, writing poetry. I am graduating this year from an Open University degree.

(Allen 2010)

In the face of the prejudice, discrimination and exclusion that typically accompany mental health challenges, it is perhaps unsurprising that too many people become 'I used to be …' people (Mudie 2011) with a present defined only in relation to mental health services and no future. 'I used to be a mother, a university student, a plumber … now I am just a mental patient'.

What do we mean by 'recovery'?

The challenge of recovery lies in finding a life and an identity beyond that of patient-hood.

[Recovery is] a way of living a satisfying, hopeful and contributing life even within the limitations caused by illness … a deeply personal, unique process of changing one's attitudes, values, feelings, goals, skills and roles … the development of new meaning and purpose in one's life as one grows beyond the catastrophic effects of mental illness.

(Anthony 1993)

Recovery is a process of healing … of adjusting one's attitudes, feelings, perceptions, beliefs, roles and goals in life. It is a painful process, yet often one of self-discovery, self-renewal and transformation. Recovery is a deeply emotional process. Recovery involves creating a new personal vision for one's self.

(Spaniol et al. 1997)

Recovery to me is not only coming to terms with what has happened in my life, the dark side of me and the things I have done, but having grown as an individual because of my experiences. Focusing on this experience as a source of growth has been the source of inspiration for recovery. I can now look back in time and know that everything that happened helped me to become the person I am today.

(Reeves 1998)

Recovery involves building a new sense of self, meaning and purpose in life; growing within and beyond what has happened. Recovery is about living hopefully – believing in the possibility of a decent present and future for yourself. It is about making sense of what has happened and getting back into the driving seat of your life (Deegan 1993). It is about recognizing your own resources and resourcefulness and using these to take back control over your life, explore your own destiny, and determine what support you may need to pursue your dreams and ambitions.

Reflective Exercise 5.1

Recovery is often best understood in relation to personal experiences. Identify a difficult experience of your own (for example: failing a driving test or bereavement, illness, unemployment). Consider your feelings at the time and how they have changed since; how your values and life view were affected (for example: major life events can lead to appreciation of everyday experiences, bereavement can lead to reassessment of personal goals, failing an exam might make you think about alternative career options, an illness might give you new ideas about helping others in similar situations).

Recovery is not about 'going back' to how things were before. All life experiences change us and change the course of our lives. Mental health challenges are no different. We cannot turn the clock back or rewrite history, but we can find a way forward. We can recover a present beyond 'mental patient' and a future beyond mental health services. The journey of recovery is a journey of discovery:

- Discovering ways of understanding and making sense of what has happened.
- Discovering that you are more – much more – than your mental health problems.
- Discovering that you are the expert.
- Discovering that you don't need to rely on services and professionals.
- Discovering that your journey continues after services deem you to be better and no longer in need of their support.
- Discovering what you can gain from, and how you can grow as a result of, the things that have happened.

I have often asked myself whether, given the choice, I would choose to have manic depressive illness ... Strangely enough I think I would choose to have it. It's complicated. Depression is awful beyond words or sounds or images ... So why would I want anything to do with this illness? Because I honestly believe that as a result of it I have felt more things, more deeply; had more experiences, more intensely; loved more, and been loved; laughed more often for having cried more often; appreciated more the springs, for all the winters; worn death 'as close as dungarees', appreciated it – and life – more; seen the finest and the most terrible in people, and slowly learned the values of caring, loyalty and seeing things through.

(Jamison 1995)

This is not an easy task. It takes great courage and determination in the face of what can seem like insurmountable odds. Odds that might cause many of us to give up.

When I first went in I felt hopeless, I was lost ... I thought it was the end of my world.

(Allen 2010)

You have the wondrously terrifying task of becoming who you are called to be ...
Your life and dreams may have been shattered – but from such ruins you can build
a new life full of value and purpose.

(Deegan 1993)

Reflective Exercise 5.2

Think back to your experience and consider when the initial shock, grief, devastation – negative feelings – began to change:

- What, if anything, stopped this happening sooner?
- If things have not improved, why not?
- What helped?
- Who helped and how?

Sadly, the courage and strength that it takes to overcome the implications of being diagnosed as mentally ill are not recognized or celebrated. The person with cancer who runs marathons is a hero, as is the amputee who climbs Everest. Instead of being seen as brave and strong, those who face up to mental health challenges are too often deemed weak and fragile.

Most people experience major mental health problems as frightening, desolate and
even destructive. The pain of madness is probably on a par with major grief, torture,
surviving Gallipoli, or being falsely accused of a serious crime. There's a big difference
though: these other experiences have legitimacy ... Though they are not well understood
by the majority, surviving them is often regarded as admirable or heroic. Madness,
however, is met with pity, fear and reproach. It does not have status as a full human
experience, and this has provided justification for cruelty, segregation and control.

(O'Hagan 2007)

Many of the challenges faced by people with mental health problems arise not from 'symptoms' or supposed personal failings but from the way in which 'the mentally ill' are so often excluded from society:

the inter-locking and mutually compounding problems of impairment,
discrimination, diminished social role, lack of economic and social participation
and disability. Among the factors at play are lack of status, joblessness, lack of

opportunities to establish a family, small or non-existent social networks,
compounding race and other discriminations, repeated rejection and consequent
restriction of hope and expectation.

(Sayce 2000)

This process of exclusion has a negative impact on the material reality of the lives of people diagnosed with mental illness and alienates them – sets people apart – from the communities in which they live. People become 'other', 'different', 'them' not 'us'.

Out of the blue your job has gone, with it any financial security you may have had.
At a stroke, you have no purpose in life and no contact with other people. You find
yourself totally isolated from the rest of the world. No one telephones you. Much
less writes. No-one seems to care if you're alive or dead.

(Bird 2001)

For some of us, an episode of mental distress will disrupt our lives so we are pushed
out of the society in which we were fully participating. For others, the early onset of
distress will mean social exclusion throughout our adult lives, with no prospect of
training for a job or hope of a future in meaningful employment. Loneliness and
loss of self-worth lead us to believe we are useless, and so we live with this sense of
hopelessness, or far too often choose to end our lives.

(Social Exclusion Unit 2003)

Mental health challenges do not occur in a vacuum – they occur in a political, economic and social context, and it is this context that is disabling. The social model of disability long recognized in the broader disability arena is equally important in understanding the situation faced by people with mental health challenges. The cognitive and emotional impairments associated with mental health conditions are no less real than the impairments of vision or mobility, but these are not disabling in and of themselves. It is the associated discrimination and exclusion that are disabling (Sayce 2000).

Almost all the problems that people with physical disabilities face are shared by
people with psychiatric disabilities (for example, difficulties in accessing housing,
employment, and community services) ... we have grown closer to the disability
community and discovered the commonalities that we share.

(Chamberlin 1993)

The challenge of recovery is both a personal journey of discovering a new sense of self, meaning and purpose, and one of challenging the discrimination and exclusion that disable us by denying us the opportunities that all citizens have a right to expect. As in the physical world 'independent living' does not mean doing things unaided (all of us are interdependent) but having all the adjustments and support you need to do the things you want to do, and having control over that support.

All disabled people having the same choice, control and freedom as any other citizen at home, at work and as members of the community. This does not necessarily mean disabled people 'doing everything for themselves' but it does mean that any practical assistance they need should be based on their own choices and aspirations.

(Office for Disability Issues 2009)

Family and friends face the challenge of recovery

It was something like perpetual bereavement … My daughter; the person who I used to know so intimately, and who I loved and wanted to rescue more desperately than I'd ever wanted anything, was beyond my reach and everything which had seemed stable and reliable so recently was not. Her actions, emotions and discourse, and therefore my own responses, were unpredictable … My girl had become a stranger to me and I to her.

(Varley 2007)

Mental health problems have a profound impact not only on the person who experiences them, but also on those who are close to them – their family, friends and carers. It is very hard to see someone you love – a child, grandchild, partner, sibling, parent, close friend – become distressed and disturbed, behaving in ways that you don't recognize or understand. Not only do you have to make sense of what has happened and struggle to find the best way of helping them, but also you have to juggle all your existing responsibilities and roles. On top of this it can be hard to navigate an array of different services and professionals who may not understand or recognize your concerns. Then there is the issue of what to say to curious friends and neighbours who may shun you, or treat you differently, because of the prejudice that surrounds mental health challenges.

What is often forgotten by people who provide services is just how important family, friends and carers are. For us all, it is the people around us, not specialized services, who provide the vast majority of social, practical and emotional support; and this is not different for people with mental health problems. Recovery is supported, facilitated and enabled by family members, friends, neighbours, colleagues, employers, faith communities, fellow students and peers who share experiences of mental health problems.

Those who love and care about the person – parents, partners, children, siblings, other relatives and close friends – face the challenge of recovery (Spaniol and Zipple 1994). Indeed they face a twin challenge (Repper *et al.* 2011):

- Helping the person they love in their journey – we must never forget that the majority of help and support that people with mental health problems receive comes not from services but from relatives.

- Keeping themselves well, rebuilding their own lives in the changed circumstances they face, finding new sources of value and meaning in their loved one and in their relationship with them.

> ## Reflective Exercise 5.3
>
> Families and friends repeatedly make a plea for more respect, recognition and information from services; rarely do they find services that both provide them with support and value their concerns for the person and understandings of the person. Consider your own feelings about working with 'carers' and list these so that all can see. Follow this with another question: If your mother, sister, child or spouse were to experience mental health problems, and be admitted to an acute inpatient unit, what sort of support would you want for yourself? How would you ask for this? How would you behave if you felt that staff did not listen to you or acknowledge your role in the person's life?

The origin of ideas about recovery

Ideas about recovery were not born from learned academics and professionals but emerged from the experience and writing of people who had themselves faced the challenge of living with a mental health condition. They can be traced back to the civil rights movement and are epitomized by Judi Chamberlin's work *On Our Own*, first published in 1977. This ground-breaking text, and many that have followed it, demonstrates that people with mental health conditions can individually and collectively find their own solutions to the challenges they face. The foundations of our understanding of recovery are the real-life recovery stories of people who have lived with and grown beyond the mental health challenges they face.

As mental health services have taken on ideas about recovery, professionals have sought its origins and development in terms of services rather than the individual journeys of the individuals whom they served. For example, Davidson *et al.* (2010) trace the roots of the 'recovery movement' in psychiatry to the 'traitement moral' pioneered by Pinel and Pussin and services such as the York Retreat. Prompted by the death of a young Friend – Hannah Mills – in the harsh and brutal York Asylum, the religious Society of Friends (Quakers) established the retreat in 1796, under the direction of William Tuke. Respect, kindness, a liberal and nourishing diet – a glass of porter ('always avoiding, in all cases, any degree of intoxication') – occupation and friendship replaced the chains, shackles, intimidation and neglect of the traditional asylum (Tuke 1813, p. 53). However, this development of what might be called 'humanitarian psychiatry' continues to place mental health services and the workers who inhabit them at centre stage. It continues to think about 'the patient in our services' rather than 'the person in their life'. The focus remains what services do to put right that which has gone wrong rather than thinking about supporting people to use their own resources to do the things they want to do.

Since the mid-1990s it has become widely accepted that the principles of recovery should underpin practice in mental health services. Since such initiatives were first made in the USA (Anthony 1993) they have spread throughout the 'developed' world. In the UK they have been reflected in the mental health strategies across the political spectrum (Department of Health (DH) 2011; The Scottish Executive 2009; Welsh Assembly Government 2005).

In the journey from civil rights activists with lived experience of mental health conditions to mainstream mental health policy there has been a tendency for mental health services to 'take over' ideas about recovery, and understand the concept in terms with which they are familiar: as a model and intervention designed to fix people or get rid of their problems. This distortion from individual journey to professional intervention has led some people to reject the whole idea of recovery.

What helps people in their recovery journey?

It is both the accounts of people facing the challenge of mental health conditions and the accounts of those who are close to them that provide us with the source materials about what is helpful in their recovery journey. If services are truly to recognize the expertise of lived experience and develop services that support people in their journeys then it is these accounts that must guide us.

Treatment, therapy and the desire to be free of debilitating symptoms are only part of the story. Most accounts place at least as much emphasis on the importance of decent lives and, relationships – recognizing and building on strengths rather than eliminating deficits and dysfunctions.

> safe, pleasant and affordable housing, well paying and fulfilling jobs ... to be treated with dignity and respect, to have control over their lives and to have genuine choices. They want to feel good about themselves and have the opportunity to achieve things that all of us do.
>
> (Bond 1994)

> I do not believe these changes came about because of the tendency for schizophrenia to improve over the years. Nor do I believe that the newer medications played a role ... David's changes came about rather quickly when professionals and family members began to focus on his considerable strengths instead of his illness. In the old days the emphasis on his treatment, aside from medication was put on helping with his abysmal 'daily living skills' – helping him learn to ride the buses, to take a shower, to make eye contact and so on. But where should he go on the bus? For whom should he have a shower? With whom should he make eye contact? ... This approach got nowhere. A few years ago ... the psychiatrist said 'I don't want to hear all that again. That's his illness, and we have not been able to change that for years. Tell me about his strengths; we would do better to work on those' ... Once a conscious effort was put into his strengths, the turnabout was dramatic.
>
> (Wasow 2001)

There are often differences in the priorities of mental health workers and people with lived experience of mental health challenges (Shepherd *et al.* 1995). While staff place greatest emphasis on the treatment, support and monitoring that professionals provide, the people whom they serve emphasize assistance in accommodating and finding meaning in their distress; support with housing, finance, social networks and physical health. Research into 'strategies for living' conducted by people with lived experience (Faulkner and Layzell 2000) found a number of different factors to be helpful in recovery:

- Acceptance
- The company of others who share similar experiences
- Emotional – people being there for you
- Finding a reason for living
- Discovering meaning and purpose in life
- Peace of mind and relaxation
- Taking control and having choices
- Security and safety
- Pleasurable things to do.

Deegan (1996) emphasizes the loss, grief and mourning that accompany mental illness and the devastating hopelessness that ensues.

> *One by one our dreams and hopes were crushed. We seemed to lose everything. We felt abandoned in our ever deepening winter ... For those of us who have been diagnosed with mental illness and who have lived in the sometimes desolate wastelands of mental health programs and institutions, hope is not just a nice sounding euphemism. It is a matter of life and death.*
>
> (*Deegan 1996*)

Chamberlin (1993) identifies three important elements which promote recovery:

- *Hope*: the belief that tomorrow can be different from today.
- *Contact with other people*: someone who believes in you even when you do not believe in yourself.
- *Positive role models:* others who have recovered.

Similarly, Ashcraft and Anthony (2005) emphasize the importance of hope and add to this a recovery environment, empowerment, choice and spirituality. While everyone's journey of recovery is unique and deeply personal, three factors repeatedly emerge as critical to recovery (Perkins 2006; Perkins and Repper 1996, 1998, 2009; Repper and Perkins 2003, 2004; Shepherd *et al.* 2008):

1. *Hope and hope-inspiring relationships*: the belief in a decent future for yourself. Not 'jolly hockey sticks' or 'pull your socks up' but that enduring sense of possibility that

arises from grieving what you have lost, finding meaning and value in your experiences and having people around you who believe in you.

2. *Taking back control over your life*: the challenges you face and the help you receive.

3. *Opportunity and participation*: the chance to do the things that you value, be a part of your communities and contribute to those communities.

Recovery: not recovering from a past, but regaining a future

Within traditional services the overarching philosophy or *raison d'être* is one of 'cure'. The primary aim is to get rid of, or at least reduce, a person's problems or symptoms. Such a philosophy guides not only the work of doctors, but also that of other professionals, although each would have a different view of the way in which difficulties, deficits or dysfunctions might best be remediated. All are essentially focused on the concept of 'moving away from' or 'freeing people from' problems or symptoms ... but moving towards what? Freeing people in order to enable them to do what?

Within such a prevailing philosophy, it is perhaps unsurprising that recovery has been viewed as yet another approach to moving away from or putting right problems. Sometimes this is reflected in a view of recovery that is essentially cure – 'recovery from symptoms'. This is reflected in accounts of recovery that stress how 'recovery' rates from different disorders have been traditionally underestimated and cite longitudinal studies which show that 'recovery' rates are higher than is typically assumed. Slade (2009), for example, cites a series of longitudinal studies of 'recovery' from schizophrenia, indicating that over half of those with the diagnosis 'recovered' completely from their symptoms and were free of medication.

Such arguments may be useful in counteracting the therapeutic pessimism that too often abounds within mental health services. Typically, within mental health services both practitioners and people with mental health conditions only see people when they are at their most distressed and most disturbed by their difficulties, and only continue to see those whose challenges persist. These longer term studies serve to remind us that there are many more people who are not visible to professionals and going about their lives without the need for services.

In his critique of the concept of recovery, Pilgrim (2008) describes it as a 'polyvalent' concept attempting to achieve an uneasy consensus between traditionally discordant groups in the service of political and economic imperatives of reducing people's reliance on services at the same time as minimizing the risks they pose to others. He argues that traditional biomedical psychiatry talks of 'recovery from illness' (recovery as the outcome of successful treatment) while social psychiatry talks of 'recovery from impairment' (recovery as the outcome of successful rehabilitation) and dissenting service users talk about 'recovery from invalidation' (recovery as the outcome of successful survival from an oppressive system). In a similar vein, Aslan (2010) defines recovery as freedom from medication and mental health services – ceasing to be a 'service user'.

I have recovered to the point that any of us in society can be. I don't need medication, and I do not need workers. I am not a service user ... I am thriving.

(Aslan 2010)

Aslan supports the notion of 'thriving' rather than 'recovery'; and only when a person does not use psychiatric medication and mental health services can they be said to be thriving. This begs the question, what about those whose problems do persist? Are there some people for whom recovery is impossible? Is it impossible for those of us who continue to use medication to move beyond mere survival and thrive?

Both Aslan (2010) and Pilgrim (2008) are continuing to frame recovery within the traditional 'cure'/'problem removal' paradigm of traditional psychiatry. You have only 'recovered' if you have 'got better' or 'moved away from services/treatments'. This is very different from the understanding of recovery espoused by the originators of the concept in relation to mental health. When Deegan (1993, p. 10) talks about medication, therapy, self-help, work, exercise and her relationship with God as 'measures that help me remain whole and healthy, even though I have a disability', or the New Zealand Mental Heath Commission (2009) defines recovery as 'Living positively with or without mental health problems', or when Anthony (1993, p. 11) describes recovery as 'living a satisfying, hopeful and contributing life even within the limitations caused by illness' they are talking about recovery in quite different terms.

This is not a mere semantic distinction. It has profound implications for what services do and how we evaluate success. For example, a traditional 'care plan' (Table 5.1) starts by defining 'problems' and rarely contains information about what the person wants to do. In these definitions recovery is clearly about being drawn to a future rather than being determined by a past, About 'moving towards' the life you want to lead, rather than 'moving away' from, or being free from, your problems, treatment and services.

Table 5.1 The wider implications of reconsidering a care plan as a recovery plan, rather than a problem-focused plan

	Problem/symptom-focused care	Recovery-focused care
Goal of services	Eradication of problems	Achievement of personal goals
Range of relevant interventions and support	Diagnosis-based treatment and supports, medication, therapy	Education to build on self-management skills and develop practical life skills (budgeting, job-seeking, tenancy), therapies, support to engage in community facilities and opportunities, peer support, help to develop interests, build on strengths, find hidden talents
Indicators of success	Reduction in symptoms, reduction in service use, satisfaction with services	Social networks (friends), employment/ education, housing, personal goal attainment
Role of staff	Therapists, carer	Carer, coach, supporter
Role of service user	Passive recipient	Expert in their own experience and recovery plan, co-creator of their own care, peer supporter for others

When we talk about recovery we are talking not about 'recovering from' mental health problems but 'recovery of' a satisfying, meaningful, valued and contributing life, albeit one that may be different from that which you previously led.

Recovery-focused practice requires quite a different approach. In order to help someone to get somewhere we need to understand where they want to go, the resources they have to help them get there and how they would like to travel. 'Effectiveness', 'outcome' and 'success' cannot be evaluated in traditional terms – like symptom reduction or discharge from services; rather achievement should be assessed in terms of personal goals and success in building up a life outside services. Although it will always be questionable how much of these achievements can be attributed to the services received, at the very least recovery-focused services must focus on enabling people to achieve such successes rather than potentially deprive them of whole lives in the pursuit of freedom from symptoms.

Recovery: conceptions and misconceptions

Confusion about what is meant by the term 'recovery' makes it important to be clear about what recovery is and what it is not (see Anthony 1993). When we talk about 'recovery' we are talking about:

> the lived or real life experience of people as they accept and overcome the challenge of the disability. They experience themselves as recovering a new sense of self and of purpose within and beyond the limits of the disability.

> (Deegan 1988)

Here, Deegan is not talking about overcoming or eradicating the disability itself, but of finding ways of overcoming the challenges that it poses – through friends, religion, exercise, distraction, meditation, medication, and so on: all of many different supports and strategies that she might call on to manage experiences and perceptions.

Not a theory of the origins of mental illness

The starting point for recovery is not a theory of the origins of mental illness. It is not another aetiological theory set up in contradistinction to 'biological', 'psychological', 'social', 'biopsycho-social', 'institutionalization' or 'existential' models. These were all developed to explain how a person's problems developed on the assumption that if you knew the causes you could determine the cures. However, this logic is faulty. The way you got into a situation does not *necessarily* tell you the way out. You may have fallen to the bottom of a well, but falling certainly won't get you out! Aspirin may be very good for ameliorating headaches, but headaches are not caused by an aspirin deficit. Recovery is about moving forward in life not getting rid of problems. Ideas about recovery do not prescribe or proscribe particular theories or courses of action (drugs = bad, psychological therapy = good). It is not a question of whether a particular model or intervention is 'right' or 'wrong', or even whether it gets rid of a person's problems. Instead the question is whether the person finds the model and/or its associated interventions helpful in rebuilding the life they want. No theory makes sense to everyone: the different professionals who comprise 'multi-disciplinary teams' typically adopt different models of mental distress, as do those whom they serve. No treatment or intervention is helpful to everyone. Whether you consider the origin of your problems to lie in your biology, traumatic experiences, psychological disturbance or the ravages wrought by mental health services themselves, you still face the challenge of rebuilding a life and this is what recovery is about.

Not about cure

Recovery is not the same as 'cure'. It does not mean that all suffering has disappeared, or that all symptoms have been removed, or that functioning has been completely restored. Some problems may disappear completely, others may be ever present, and many will recur from time to time. Any traumatic experience leaves its scars, but, gradually, we can learn to accommodate it into our life – it becomes part of us and it ceases to govern every moment of our waking lives and define our possibilities. So with mental health conditions, even though challenges may persist, people can and do learn ways of accommodating these so that they interfere less with what you want to do.

> *One of the biggest lessons I have had to accept is that recovery is not the same thing as being cured. After 21 years of living with this thing it still hasn't gone away.*
>
> *(Deegan 1993)*

Not a set formula

Too often we seek protocols and procedures for dealing with particular problems. Attempts have been made to do this in terms of defining the 'stages' of the recovery process. For example, Andreason *et al.* (2006, p. 974) have defined five 'stages' of recovery beginning with 'moratorium', 'a time of withdrawal characterized by a profound sense of loss and hopelessness', progressing through 'awareness', 'preparation' and 'rebuilding' to 'growth', 'characterised by self-management of the illness, resilience and a positive sense of self.'

While such 'stages' may be identifiable from people's accounts of their own journeys, everyone's journey is unique and deeply personal (Anthony 1993). Different people start from different places, choose different paths in life and sometimes change course completely. Recovery, like life, is not a linear process: there will be set-backs and 'great leaps forward' along the way. Various versions of these 'stages' have been incorporated into 'recovery interventions' developed by professionals to assist people in their journey. For example, the 'Recovery Star' (McKeith *et al.* 2010) identifies 10 dimensions of growth (such as living skills, addictive behaviour, identity and self-esteem, responsibilities and managing mental health) with progression rated on a 10-step ladder of change taking your from 'stuck' to 'self-reliance'. While some people find such instruments helpful in their journey, they do not in and of themselves, define or constitute recovery, and other people find the language and approach alienating.

There are many dangers inherent in attempts to define the recovery journey. For example, people may be considered, or consider themselves, a 'failure' if they do not progress in the prescribed manner. There may be times in anyone's journey when withdrawal (moratorium) is useful and helpful:

> *giving up, apathy and indifference become a way of surviving and protecting the last vestiges of a wounded self.*

> *(Deegan 1990)*

Similarly, people differ in the way they choose to approach challenges. When faced with a cold swimming pool some people choose to jump in, while others prefer to gradually enter by easy stages, yet others will decide that the reward is not worth the effort and choose to do something completely different. There are no rules of recovery, no formula for 'success'. Everyone must find their own way – people do not progress neatly up a unidirectional ladder.

> *Once recovery becomes systematised, you have got it wrong. Once it has been reduced to a set of principles it is wrong. It is a unique and individualised process.*

> *(Deegan 1999)*

Not a professional intervention

Too often services and professionals believe that it is their job to fix people – put right that which has gone wrong. Whether by pharmacological, psychological, occupational or social interventions human beings cannot be fixed like you might fix a car or a washing machine.

> *Over the years I have worked hard to become an expert in my own self-care. For me, being in recovery means I don't just take medications. Just taking medications is a passive stance. Rather I use medications as part of my recovery process. In the same way, I don't just go into hospital. Just 'going into hospital' is a passive stance. Rather, I use the hospital when I need to. Over the years I have learned different ways of helping myself. Sometimes I use medications, therapy, self-help and mutual support groups, friends, my relationship with God, work, exercise, spending time in nature – all of these measures help me remain whole and healthy, even though I have a disability.*

> *(Deegan 1993)*

The essence of recovery is about helping people to recognize, develop and use their own resources, and those available to them, to grow within and beyond what has happened. These resources may include mental health treatments and supports, but mental health professionals and services do not hold the key and recovery can and does occur without specialist intervention. Warner's (2009) international review of research into recovery and schizophrenia offers a salutary lesson to those of us working in 'modern' mental health services:

> It emerges that one of the most robust findings about schizophrenia is that a substantial proportion of those who present with the illness will recover completely or with good functional capacity, with or without modern medical treatment.

> (Warner 2009)

Recovery: not 'them' and 'us'

Recovery is not something that 'they' do. It is not specific to those who face mental health challenges. It is a common human experience. We all experience what Shakespeare has called 'the slings and arrows of outrageous fortune' whether it be mental health challenges or the death of someone we love, physical illness or impairment, the end of a relationship, unemployment or redundancy, failing a key examination, trauma, abuse, etc. Traumatic and life-changing events challenge our assumptions about who we are, why we are here, what is really important to us, where we want to go and what we want from life. They offer not only heartache but also the chance to re-evaluate and change direction if we so want – not 'breakdown' but 'breakthrough'.

No human being can ever fully understand the life and experience of another, and the experience of mental health challenges and all that surround them cannot be understood by someone who has not faced them. The experience of each person facing mental health challenges is unique. But we can connect with each other not only by defining our differences, but by recognizing our common humanity and that which we share. In embracing a recovery perspective we are all on a journey of discovery.

References

Allen S (2010) (ed.) *Our Stories: Moving On, Recovery and Well-being*. London: South West London Mental Health NHS Trust – Forensic Services.

Andreason R, Caputi P, Oades L (2006) Stages of recovery instrument: Development of a measure of recovery from serious mental illness. *Australian and New Zealand Journal of Psychiatry* **40**, 972–80.

Anthony WA (1993) Recovery from mental illness: The guiding vision of the mental health system in the 1990s. *Psychosocial Rehabilitation Journal* **16**, 11–23.

Ashcraft L, Anthony WA (2005) A story of transformation. An agency fully embraces recovery. *Behavioural Healthcare Tomorrow* **14**, 12–22.

Aslan M (2010) Many service user workers are still wobbly. Online: www.psychminded. co.uk/news/news2010/jan10/Get-radical-again-in-mental-health004.html (accessed 21 February 2011).

Bird L (2001) Poverty, social exclusion and mental health: A survey of people's personal experiences. *A Life in the Day* **5**, 3.

Bond GR (1994) Psychiatric rehabilitation outcome, in The Publication Committee of IAPSRS (ed.) *An Introduction to Psychiatric Rehabilitation.* Columbia, MD: International Association of Psychosocial Rehabilitation Services, pp. 490–4.

Chamberlin J (1977) *On Our Own.* London: Mind Publications.

Chamberlin J (1993) Psychiatric disabilities and the ADA. An advocate's perspective, in Gostin LO, Beyer HA (eds) *Implementing the Americans with Disabilities Act.* Baltimore, MD: Brookes, pp. 71–9.

Davidson L, Rakfeldt J, Strauss J (2010) *The Roots of the Recovery Movement in Psychiatry. Lessons Learned.* Oxford: Wiley Blackwell.

Deegan P (1988) Recovery: The lived experience of rehabilitation. *Psychosocial Rehabilitation Journal* **11**(4), 11–19.

Deegan P (1990). Spirit breaking: When the helping professions hurt. *The Humanistic Psychologist* **18** (3), 301–13.

Deegan P (1993) Recovering our sense of value after being labeled. *Journal of Psychosocial Nursing* **31**(4), 7–11.

Deegan P (1996) Recovery as a journey of the heart. *Psychosocial Rehabilitation Journal* **19**(3), 91–7.

Deegan PE (1999) *Recovery: An Alien Concept.* Paper presented at Strangefish Conference 'Recovery: An Alien concept' at Chamberlin Hotel, Birmingham.

Department of Health (2011) *No Health Without Mental Health.* London: HMSO.

Faulkner A, Layzell S (2000) *Strategies for Living. A Report of User-Led Research into People's Strategies for Living with Mental Distress.* London: The Mental Health Foundation.

Jamison, K (1995) *An Unquiet Mind.* New York, NY: Alfred A.Knopf

McKeith J, Burns S, Onyemaechi I, Okonkwo N (2010) *The Recovery Star: User Guide*, 2nd edn. London: Mental Heath Providers Forum.

Mudie S (2011) *A Service User Perspective.* Paper presented at the Cardiff Recovery Charter Launch, City Hall, Cardiff.

New Zealand Mental Health Commission (2009) Poster '6 ways to use a recovery approach'.

Office for Disability Issues (2009) *Roadmap 2025. Achieving Disability Equality by 2005.* London: HM Government.

O'Hagan M (2007) Parting thoughts. *Mental Notes* **18**, 4–5.

Perkins R (2006) First person: 'you need hope to cope', in Roberts G, Davenport S, Holloway F, Tattan T (eds) *Enabling Recovery. The Principles and Practice of Rehabilitation Psychiatry.* London: Gaskell, pp. 112–24.

Perkins RE, Repper JM (1996) *Working Alongside People with Long Term Mental Health Problems.* London: Chapman & Hall (reprinted by Stanley Thornes 1999).

Perkins RE, Repper JM (1998) *Clinical Dilemmas in Community Mental Health Practice. Choice or Control*. Oxford: Radcliffe Medical Press.

Perkins R, Repper J (2009) Rehabilitation and recovery, in Norman I, Ryrie I (ed.) *The Art and Science of Mental Health Nursing*. Slough: Open University Press.

Pilgrim D (2008) 'Recovery' and current mental health policy. *Chronic Illness* **4**(4), 295–304.

Reeves A (1998) *Recovery. A Holistic Approach*. Runcorn: Handsell Publishing.

Repper JM, Perkins RE (2003) *Social Inclusion and Recovery: A Model for Mental Health Practice*. London: Balliere Tindall.

Repper J, Perkins R (2004) Social Inclusion and acute care, in Harrison M, Howard D, Mitchell D (eds) *Acute Mental Health Nursing. From Acute Concerns to Capable Practitioner*. London: Sage.

Repper J, Perkins R, Shepherd G, Boardman J (2011) *Recovery: Rebuilding life With Mental Health Problems. A Journey of Discovery for Family, Friends and Carers*. London: Centre for Mental Health/NHS Confederation/National Mental Health Development Unit.

Sayce L (2000) *From Psychiatric Patient to Citizen*. London: Palgrave Macmillan

Shepherd G, Murray A, Muijen M (1995) Perspectives on schizophrenia: A survey of user, family care and professional views regarding effective care. *Journal of Mental Health* **4**, 403–22.

Shepherd G, Boardman J, Slade M (2008) *Making Recovery a Reality*. London: Sainsbury Centre for Mental Health.

Slade M (2009) *Personal Recovery and Mental Illness*. Cambridge: Cambridge University Press.

Social Exclusion Unit (2003) *Mental Health and Social Exclusion*. London: Office of the Deputy Prime Minister, Social Exclusion Unit.

Spaniol L, Zipple A (1994) Coping strategies for families of people who have a mental illness, in Lefley H, Wasow M (eds) *Helping Families Cope with Mental Illness*. New York, NY: Guilford Press, pp. 178–90.

Spaniol L, Gagne C, Koehler M (1997) Recovery from serious mental illness: What it is and how to assist people in their recovery. *Continuum* **4**(4), 3–15.

The Scottish Executive (2009) *Towards a Mentally Flourishing Scotland: The Future of Mental Health Improvement in Scotland 2008–2001*. Edinburgh: The Scottish Executive.

Tuke S (1813) *A Description of The Retreat. An Institution Near York, for Insane Persons of The Society of Friends*. York: W Alexander.

Varley J (2007) Frustrated and angry, Chapter 12, in Hardcastle M, Kennard D, Grandison S, Hardcastle M, Kennard D, Grandison S, Fagin L (eds) *Experiences of Mental Health Inpatient Care. Narratives from Service Users, Carers and Professionals*. London: Routledge.

Warner R (2009) Recovery from schizophrenia and the recovery model. *Current Opinion in Psychiatry* **22**, 374–80.

Wasow M (2001) Strengths versus deficits, or musician versus schizophrenic. *Psychiatric Services* **52**, 1306–7.

Welsh Assembly Government (2005) *Raising the Standard: The Revised Adult Mental Health National Service Framework and Action Plan for Wales*. Cardiff: Welsh Assembly Government.

Part 2

The Policy and Organizational Context of Mental Health Care

CHAPTER SIX

Stephen Tee and **Judith A Lathlean**

Appraising and using evidence in mental health practice

Learning outcomes

- Be able to conduct an effective systematic search of literature relevant to mental health practice and appraise the evidence emanating from research and other sources
- Be able to consider and discuss ethical and/or governance implications that arise in the use of evidence
- Be able to interpret findings taking into account limitations and challenges of the implementation of evidence-based practice

Introduction

In previous chapters you were introduced to psychological theories that can help you improve your self-awareness and practice. You were also introduced to the values-based approaches that aim to improve your understanding of personal and professional values, as well as consider concepts such as recovery and thriving. This chapter will now help you develop skills in appraising and using evidence within your everyday mental health practice. It is intended as a user-friendly approach to developing the skills required for delivering evidence-based practice. It uses a case example to explore the origins, nature and purpose of evidence and its value in achieving best practice. The chapter also integrates service user perspectives in order to best represent the experiences and needs of those who access mental health services.

Using an evidence-based practice framework, the chapter will help you develop the skills required to identify, appraise and implement evidence in practice. In doing so, it aims to help you achieve one of the cornerstones of being an effective health care professional, namely the considered and critical use of contemporary best practice. Completing the reflective exercises within this chapter will also help you achieve the following competency as detailed in the Nursing and Midwifery Council's (NMC) standards for pre-registration in nursing:

> *All nurses must use up-to-date knowledge and evidence to assess, plan, deliver and evaluate care, communicate findings, influence change and promote health and best practice.*
>
> *(NMC 2010)*

So why is being able to appraise and use evidence important?

Practitioners involved in the delivery of health care practice are required to ensure that interventions are based on the best available evidence. But what constitutes 'best evidence'? How do you find evidence and assess its value? How do you use evidence in practice? What barriers might you encounter in using evidence? What about the service users' preferences? Chapter 3 explored how values-based approaches can be used to take account of individual perspectives, and in this chapter we will hopefully provide some additional answers to questions that typically arise when notions of evidence in practice are first encountered.

Nursing's move in 2013 towards an all-graduate profession at entry has meant a re-examination of the skills required to be an effective practitioner. A key graduate attribute is the ability to be able to use and apply evidence drawn from clinical research. Developments in mental health nursing practice over the past two decades have seen a shift from focusing purely on tasks where everything is broken down into fixed routines to a more holistic approach, in which care and treatment are delivered in a person-centred, individualized manner. This simple shift requires a different set of skills to work collaboratively with an individual, assess their particular needs and carry out procedures or treatments in a culturally sensitive and professional manner.

However, this is not the whole story because we can work in a holistic manner and still deliver interventions based on evidence and procedures that are either ineffective or, at worse, harmful. Achieving best practice requires practitioners to approach the delivery of care with a sophisticated skills-set that enables them to assess individual needs and preferences, while being cognizant of the legal and professional requirements of practice. They also need to be able to select, appraise and use research and other sources of evidence in their everyday practice.

The shift in nursing towards all-graduate status emphasizes the need for practitioners to develop strategies for first selecting appropriate and relevant information from a wide range of professional and inter-professional sources of knowledge. Second, they need to critically appraise the information in order to gain a coherent and evidence-based understanding of practice. Only through the development of these skills will nurses be able provide the most effective care based on the best available evidence. For instance, consider Case Study 6.1.

> **Case Study 6.1**
>
> Since working in a mental health acute admissions unit you have encountered several service users who appear distant and difficult to engage in conversation or activity. At times they present as withdrawn and pre-occupied. You want to help but are not sure of the best approach. However, you are aware from the literature that there is research that explores this issue. What evidence would you draw on to support your approach to helping this group of people?

In order to answer the question in Case Study 6.1 the first step is to consider where we can obtain evidence, so that we can decide what we might do to best help.

Theoretical background

McKenna (2009) provides an excellent discussion on the nature of evidence, drawing on theories of rationalism, empiricism, historicism, aesthetics and ethics. The key messages are that evidence can be derived from reason (rationalism), rigorous observation and measurement (empiricism), experience (historicism), tacit knowledge and intuition (aesthetics) and notions of right and wrong (ethics). These ideas are reflected in the frameworks that guide practice. The NMC's Professional Code (2008) is underpinned by a deontological ethical approach of protecting the rights of the individual. These ethical principles are:

1. Respect for the person (which is known as autonomy)

2. A responsibility to treat everyone equally and ensure that they are informed of their rights (which is known as justice)

3. An obligation that decisions taken maximize benefit (known as beneficence)

4. An obligation to avoid harm and keep people safe (known as non-maleficence).

Therefore in order to practise in a safe, proficient and effective way, the decisions and judgements made by a nurse need to be underpinned by a set of professional values developed from sound ethical principles and articulated through a sound process of reasoning. Working within this framework, a nurse will develop confidence in their decision-making and, through increasing experience and reflection, be able to develop their ethical reasoning skills.

Case Study 6.1

Continued

Our professional obligations require us to respect individual autonomy; in other words, to behave in a way that allows individuals to participate in decision-making and to consent to all aspects of treatment and care. We must treat everyone equally and approach them in a non-judgemental manner while respecting their values and beliefs. We must also ensure that our interventions are helpful and do not cause additional harm or distress. But how do we know whether our interventions are beneficial or harmful?

Delivering high standards of care based on best evidence

The delivery of high-quality care is captured in the third element of the NMC Code that emphasizes notions of evidence, skills, knowledge and standards of practice. As a nurse you are expected to provide care based on the best available evidence, keep your skills up to date and maintain accurate records. While the bedrock of professional practice is to make decisions based on sound ethical principles you need also to exercise sound judgement as to what constitutes best evidence. At one level this may appear straightforward, by simply following best practice guidelines. But evidence is constantly evolving and changing; and as practitioners we have access to a plethora of studies, theoretical papers, guidelines, discussion documents and, importantly, considerable literature written by service users from which we are expected to judge the best way to intervene or carry out a procedure.

Returning to McKenna's discussion about the nature of evidence, the focus of this chapter is to support you in developing the skills of judging the value and use of rigorous evidence in practice, in other words 'empiricism'. This focus is not intended to minimize the value of other forms of evidence, which are addressed in other chapters, but will develop your ability to discern between strong and weak evidence, so that, as a qualified practitioner, you can integrate research evidence within your clinical decision-making. We will of course draw on experience (historicism) to make clinical judgements, but we again must exercise care; just because we have always approached something in a certain way does not make it right to continue if there is rigorous empirical evidence to support a different approach. Sometimes the culture of practice means things are done unquestioningly in certain ways but we need to have the courage to question practice and consider alternatives. Equally, tacit knowledge and intuition (aesthetics) are important tools for the experienced nurse working in difficult and pressurized situations, but we must, through constant reflection, question the judgements we are making so that we do not fall into a similar trap of discounting contrary approaches or evidence.

Working within a clinical environment, employing organizations will have established frameworks, policies and procedures to monitor standards of care and treatment. So although there is an individual professional responsibility to ensure practice is based on contemporary evidence and sound ethical principles, the organization will also need to satisfy itself that safe and effective processes are being followed. This area of monitoring is known as governance. External bodies such as the Care Quality Commission (CQC 2011) check the quality of services and investigate specific issues; they will look at practice and benchmark this against policies and procedures and, in doing so, it becomes public knowledge.

The value of clinical governance to support decisions

Governance is an important component of the decision-making landscape for nurses. Clinical governance is a framework used to examine potential causes of failure and to take preventive action in order to avoid risk or damage to individuals. The governance frameworks, instigated by employers, seek to ensure that care is delivered to appropriate standards. Storey and Buchanan (2008) suggest that governance represents a cultural shift from provider-oriented services to service-user-oriented services. It provides a system of accountability and aims to ensure:

- Transparency around responsibility and accountability
- Effective quality improvement systems, which includes the application of evidence-based practice
- Plans for education and training
- Risk management plans
- Clear and integrated procedures to identify and remedy poor performance.

Organizations, such as National Health Service (NHS) Trusts, will use a system of processes including audit, clinical effectiveness, continuing professional development, patient and public involvement, performance management and risk management to gather a clear picture of the quality of the care and treatment. These are important considerations for nurses who will be expected to make a significant contribution to each clinical governance component. As indicated earlier in the chapter, when considering accountability, nurses will have dual responsibilities and accountabilities to both their professional body and their employer. The system of clinical governance highlights those aspects that will ensure the nurse is making an effective contribution to the quality of care within the employing organization.

Using evidence

The implications of this are that nurses have professional, legal and contractual obligations to ensure that clinical decisions and care procedures are based on the best available evidence and conform to contemporary standards of practice. Further it highlights that evidence-based decision-making is dynamic, in that it is changing and evolving in response to emerging new research, changing laws and the emergence or extension of new practice roles. The chief skills for nurses to master are to be able to draw critically on sources of knowledge and judge what is the most appropriate approach for each unique situation.

Case Study 6.1

Continued

We know there is literature, drawn from a predominantly psychotherapeutic perspective (see Chapter 2), on the therapeutic use of self, therapeutic communication and in particular the dynamics of relationships (for examples see Barker 2009; Ersser 1997; Freshwater 2002). However, we need the skills to evaluate the strength of this evidence before we employ it in our practice.

Evidence-based practice

A contemporary approach to using evidence is encapsulated in the term evidence-based practice, which is defined by Sackett and colleagues (1996) as:

> *the conscientious, explicit, and judicious use of current best evidence in making decisions about the care of individual patients … [by] integrating individual clinical expertise with the best available external clinical evidence from systematic research.*
>
> *(p. 71)*

It can be seen that this definition places an emphasis on the nurse needing to exercise judgement in the care they deliver in order to discern between effective or ineffective approaches. When applied to evidence, the nurse will need skills in determining the quality of the evidence to support the decision being made. The definition emphasizes two important elements, namely clinical expertise (historicism and aesthetics) and systematic research (empiricism). It is therefore not considered sufficient to continually draw on expertise if this is not fully informed by the latest research in a particular area of practice.

So how do you decide what is good evidence? A helpful starting point is to consider the hierarchy of evidence constructed by Muir Gray (2001), which identifies the strength of evidence based on the type of research method employed (Table 6.1).

Table 6.1 The hierarchy of evidence

Type	Evidence
I	Strong evidence from at least one systematic review of multiple, well-designed, randomized controlled trials
II	Strong evidence from at least one properly designed, randomized controlled trial of appropriate size
III	Evidence from well-designed trials without randomization, single group pre–post cohort, time series or matched case–control studies
IV	Evidence from well-designed non-experimental studies from more than one centre or research group
V	Opinions of respected authorities, based on clinical evidence, descriptive studies or reports of expert committees

It can be seen that, according to Muir Gray, the strongest evidence is that derived from a systematic review of multiple randomized controlled trials that have been well designed. This hierarchy suggests that nurses should seek to use evidence from higher up the hierarchy when making decisions and delivering care. However, problems arise when strong evidence is not there. The problem, according to Dollaghan (2004), is that systematic reviews often get more attention in the literature than smaller qualitative studies that may be of equal value. This deference to science is explored in more detail in Chapter 9. In areas such as mental health, large systematic reviews may not be possible or may not have been funded, and so other forms of evidence are required to inform the nurse's practice and decision-making. Similarly, randomized controlled trials are not suited to addressing questions about 'how' and in what ways things are related.

It could be argued that in complex areas of practice, such as mental health, there is demand for even greater skill in analysing, interpreting and implementing evidence from wider sources than in those areas of practice where systematic reviews are commonly conducted. The mental health nurse needs to be aware of, and draw from all levels of, the hierarchy of evidence to keep abreast of developments in the field. This includes developments in the voluntary sector and user-led alternatives. Having considered the nature of evidence the next step is to consider how to explore the evidence. To focus this activity it is helpful to have a question from practice that you want to answer.

Framing and reframing original questions arising from critical reflection on practice

From your experience in practice you are aware that there is evidence to support particular approaches to working with individuals who are difficult to engage but you are not sure how to find the evidence or evaluate the strength of that evidence. Therefore a helpful approach is to frame an appropriate question. Framing a question is arguably the most important element in the process, as it will guide your search strategy, the evidence you choose and the resulting decision you make about care. If your question is too loose or woolly you will find yourself overwhelmed with evidence.

A helpful acronym that can support the development of a question is PICO (Schardt *et al.* 2007).

Patient/ person/problem (P); Intervention (I); Control or comparison (C); and Outcome (O).

Translating this to the problem above we get:

P = Adult individuals who are difficult to engage/social isolation and withdrawal due to mental health problems

I = Therapeutic communication

C = Non-intervention

O = Improved social engagement and reduced withdrawal.

A possible question could therefore be: Can therapeutic communication approaches, for adults experiencing social isolation and withdrawal due to mental health problems, lead to improved social engagement and reduced withdrawal, when compared with non-intervention?

Reflective Exercise 6.1

Try creating a question using an example of a problem you have encountered in practice.

Below are some further examples of research questions developed using the PICO framework. As you can see there are several ways of structuring an effective question:

- What components of targeted dementia (P) care education and training for clinical staff (I) lead to improvements in the standards of patient care (O), when compared with usual care (C)?

- Do individuals who have been brought up in families where there is problem drinking (I) have a greater risk (O) of developing alcoholism (P), when compared with normal populations (C)?

- Is dialectical behavioural therapy (I) an effective therapeutic approach (O) in the care of individuals with challenging behaviours (P), when compared with treatment as usual (C)?

- What are the components of an effective observation policy (I) that reduces risk (O) in individuals demonstrating suicidal behaviours (P), compared with normal care (C)?

- Does service user involvement (I) in clinical decision-making (P) lead to improvements in mental health care (O), when compared with services where service user involvement does not routinely take place (C)?

Having identified the initial question, you may evolve it further, to include sub-questions. You may quickly find the answer to your question, i.e. that therapeutic communication techniques do lead to improvements in a person's social engagement, but you may then want to know the components of the therapeutic techniques and the conditions under which they were implemented. In other words are particular therapeutic techniques or orientations more effective than others. This will require a deeper analysis of the studies than just determining whether the approach was effective in terms of outcome.

Systematic searching, identification of criteria and selection of robust evidence

In order to obtain the best evidence, the nurse will need to develop the skills of identifying, selecting and appraising the available evidence. Sackett *et al.* (2000) suggest that the search for the evidence should be limited to 'high-yield' sources that are directly relevant to clinical practice, adding that sources should be contemporary and not dated. Textbooks can provide useful background reading, but the evidence within them can quickly become dated and so databases, which are easily available through the university or health service library, are the best sources of evidence.

The challenge for you is to manage the sheer volume of evidence that is available in the public domain. One solution to this is to look at publications that provide a critique of recently published research. Whilst quick, relatively straightforward and a good starting point they are only as good as the day they were submitted for publication and can quickly become out of date. An alternative is to use databases such as the Cochrane Collaboration, MEDLINE, or CINAHL (see below). Before embarking on a search you will need to set some parameters around the search. This involves constructing inclusion and exclusion criteria, choosing appropriate databases to identify search terms.

Inclusion and exclusion criteria

Inclusion criteria identify the characteristics of the studies that you feel will most likely answer your question. Exclusion criteria identify those studies that you will reject as they do not answer your question. Table 6.2 provides an example of how inclusion and exclusion criteria can be used to focus your search and ensure that the studies collected are most likely to answer your question.

Once you have clarified your research question and inclusion and exclusion criteria it is necessary to identify the databases you will search. Examples of databases are listed below and include a brief explanation of their focus, content and potential value. This list is not intended to be exhaustive as there are many databases available depending on your research question and subject area.

Table 6.2 Inclusion and exclusion criteria

Inclusion criteria	Exclusion criteria	Rationale
Studies looking at therapeutic communication and engagement	Studies looking at therapeutic group approaches	The components of effective therapeutic interventions that increase individual client engagement are the important consideration here. While group approaches may be relevant this is not the primary focus
Studies involving participants experiencing mental health problems	Studies involving participants who are not experiencing mental health problems	The focus of the approach is to engage individuals who are experiencing mental health problems. While there may be studies looking at engagement in the context of other disorders, there are unique aspects to be considered in mental health which other studies may not address
Working age adults (18 years and over)	Children, adolescents and those below 18 years old or individuals over 65	The constraints of service structure are such that clients will fall within the age range of working age adults
Studies published in English language	Studies published in other languages that have not been translated into English	Limited access to translation services
Studies published from the year 1991 to present	Studies before 1991	The last two decades have seen considerable change in terms of service configuration, treatment and research, which would limit the value of studies before this date
Primary quantitative or qualitative studies including published literature reviews	Secondary sources	The research question could be answerable through a combination of quantitative and/or qualitative study designs

Case Study 6.1

Continued

Many clinical textbooks inform us that skilled and targeted therapeutic communication for someone experiencing isolation and withdrawal can lead to reduced isolation and increased engagement with social activities. However, to be effective we need to understand the specific components that have potentially therapeutic benefit and, perhaps more importantly, those aspects that can be potentially harmful to the therapeutic relationship with the isolated individual.

Choosing your databases

The databases available contain subject-relevant literature and university library services hold licences allowing students access to search the listings. Databases are increasingly sophisticated and contain a whole range of useful tools to help you search and locate appropriate articles. This will often include access to full print versions of articles that will make your job much easier. For the purposes of a study in mental health a typical search will include the databases described below. NHS Trusts often provide access to these databases, and have a research and development (R&D) department from which advice can be sought.

Cochrane database

The Cochrane Collaboration (www.cochrane.org/glossary/5#term159) was established in 1993 and prepares, updates and promotes the accessibility of Cochrane reviews, with over 4000 published online. Cochrane reviews are systematic reviews produced by people working in health care to identify the best available evidence. One example of a review in mental health is that conducted by Malone *et al.* (2007), who sought to determine the effectiveness of community mental health teams. Another review by Duncan *et al.* (2010) looked at whether shared decision-making for people with mental health conditions improved outcomes.

PsycINFO

The PsycINFO (www.apa.org/pubs/databases/psycinfo/index.aspx) database provides extensive and systematic coverage of the psychological literature from the 1800s to the present day. It has careful and precise indexing and includes bibliographic citations, abstracts, cited references and descriptive information to enable you to identify what you need easily. It focuses on the behavioural and social sciences.

CINAHL

The Cumulative Index to Nursing and Allied Health Literature (CINAHL; www.cinahl. com) is considered the most authoritative resource for nursing and allied health professionals. It provides an index of around 3000 journals and contains 2 000 000 records dating back to the early 1980s.

MEDLINE

MEDLINE (www.medline.cos.com) is the National Library of Medicine's bibliographic database and covers the fields of medicine, nursing and the health care system. It indexes 4800 current biomedical journals.

PsycArticles

The PsycArticles database (www.apa.org/pubs/databases/psycarticles/index.aspx) provides 150 000 full-text, peer-reviewed scholarly and scientific articles in psychology.

Ovid

The Ovid database (www.gateway.ovid.com/autologin.html) contains 1200 peer-reviewed journals covering a range of scientific, medical and health care disciplines, including nursing, allied health, psychology and psychiatry.

NICE

The National Institute for Health and Clinical Excellence (NICE; www.nice.org.uk) provides up-to-date guidance and best practice on a whole range of clinical problems. It is a UK organization responsible for providing national guidance on promoting good health and preventing and treating ill health. There is an emphasis for NHS Trusts to follow this guidance, and the CQC often audits this requirement.

NHS Evidence

NHS Evidence (www.evidence.nhs.uk) is a gateway to good practice information from various sources. It is free and encouraged by service providers.

Social Care Online

Another good example is Social Care Online (www.scie-socialcareonline.org.uk). This is more focused on social care but is going to be working with NICE more closely in the future on common health issues, so NICE guidance will become less medically focused in some areas.

Reflective Exercise 6.2

Search skills will prove to be very useful for all your academic written and clinical work so spend an hour or more exploring these sites and becoming familiar with the functions and scope of each database. Develop your skills by inserting, adding and refining search terms. Read the following section to help you develop your searching skills.

Identifying search terms

Search terms can be used individually or in combination to refine and focus your search. There are two types of search term: controlled, which relate to the subject itself, and non-controlled, which include synonyms and acronyms. An example of a controlled term is 'therapeutic communication'.

Search terms can be broken down as follows:

- Approaches: therapeutic communication, therapeutic relationships, dynamics, engagement
- Symptoms/diagnosis: isolation, withdrawal, preoccupation
- Client group: adults, working-age, inpatients.

Boolean operators are used to connect terms. These include the words AND, OR and NOT. By inserting these connectors between terms you will link descriptors and narrow or expand your search. So, for example, 'therapeutic communication' could be linked to 'withdrawal' and 'isolation'. This will enable you to retrieve articles that contain all three terms. You will need to repeat several searches, each time connecting and narrowing your search, to ensure you achieve a broad and thorough search of the literature at that point in time.

As you become more practised, you will be able to speed up your search and, by reading the abstracts of articles available online, include or exclude appropriate articles. The aim of your search is to end up with a list of articles and their abstracts that can be more thoroughly analysed to determine their value in answering your question.

Critically appraising the evidence

Now that you have your articles, the next stage is to appraise them. Critical appraisal is the process of critically reading an article. You may have found a paper that appears to answer your question but you cannot take it at face value. This is because, although many articles are published in what seem to be 'eminent' journals, the scientific quality of the papers can vary enormously. It is therefore important to be able to identify the rigour of the research process and the validity of the data to determine whether the conclusions drawn are based on sound knowledge; and that subsequent decisions you may make are the best in the light of what is currently known about the subject.

Critical appraisal is therefore a skill that will enable you to assess the articles you have chosen and, like any skill, it takes a little practice before you perfect the technique. However, once you have mastered the skill you will be able to quickly exclude poor quality studies and choose those that have sufficient value.

Critical appraisal essentially involves three steps or questions. First, are the results trustworthy? Second, do the results show any differences, changes, benefits or outcomes? And third, are the results relevant and applicable to the situation? This might sound complicated, but there are a number of useful tools to help with this. Unfortunately, one tool does not fit all and it is necessary to look at the type of study in terms of design. Typically the study will be one of the following:

- Systematic review
- Randomized controlled trial
- Qualitative research
- Economic evaluation study
- Cohort study
- Case–control study
- Diagnostic test study.

You can find suitable appraisal tools at the following websites, and which are free to download for personal use:

- Critical Appraisal Skills Programme: www.sph.nhs.uk/what-we-do/public-health-workforce/resources/critical-appraisals-skills-programme
- Casp-birmingham.org: www.casp-birmingham.org/

The above CASP tools aim to enable you to develop the skills to find and make sense of the research evidence you have chosen from your search; in other words helping you to translate knowledge into practice. There are also training workshops available to help you with this process. Once you have chosen the tool, it is then a matter of working through the process.

A challenge for practitioners working in mental health is that much of the available evidence is predicated on a medical view of 'mental illness' and may not address the sort of questions that are important to a mental health nurse. There are often few studies that employ methods at the top end of the hierarchy of evidence and so practice is reliant on evidence drawn from expert opinion published in respected, high-impact journals and consequently it becomes even more difficult to evaluate the quality of evidence available. A typical search for 'therapeutic communication' might throw up the following article:

Burnard P (2003) Ordinary chat and therapeutic conversation: phatic communication and mental health nursing, published Journal of Psychiatric and Mental Health Nursing **10** *(6), 678–82.*

It seems to address your question, is written by a respected authority in the field and is published in a reputable journal. It is not immediately apparent from the abstract whether the article is quantitative or qualitative in design or a summary of previous studies and discussion on the current state of the art. Further reading of the complete paper is required to determine the type of tool to use.

The qualitative tool located in the CASP source above includes 10 questions to help you make sense of the research and seeks to address the rigour, credibility and relevance of the research. The choice of quantitative tool is made more complex by the fact that you will need to identify the study design. Is it a case–control, cohort or randomized controlled trial type of study? Once this is established this will guide your choice of tool. Each of these quantitative tools asks a similar question around the validity and applicability of the results.

Other issues to consider

When considering evidence it is important to be careful about the use of basic scientific findings. Whilst they may seem to provide the 'strongest' form of evidence, in terms of rigour, if the studies were conducted in unrealistically controlled conditions, you will need to consider their relevance to the real world of practice. Often such studies will need to be followed by studies focused on the realities of clinical practice to determine their applicability.

The NMC Professional Code (NMC 2008) requires nurses to question evidence and use contemporary sources of evidence, rather than relying on textbooks, which can become out of date owing to policy, treatment and legislative changes. Textbooks such as this can help provide some of the tools for implementing evidence but it will be down to you to find and assess the value of the most up-to-date sources of evidence.

Does the evidence answer your research question?

Accurate and skilful critical appraisal of the evidence will then allow you to determine whether there is sufficient and robust evidence to answer your question. Invariably there may remain questions over the evidence, but it will be down to your clinical judgement to decide whether the evidence is strong enough to support a change of practice. In the case of the question raised in Case Study 6.1:

> *Can therapeutic communication approaches, for adults experiencing social isolation and withdrawal due to mental health problems, lead to improved social engagement and reduced withdrawal, when compared with non-intervention?*

You may find that there is evidence to support the use of therapeutic communication for people who are withdrawn and isolated as a result of mental health problems. After having appraised the evidence you may have been able to determine the specific components of therapeutic communication that optimize effectiveness in different contexts.

However, ethical practice dictates that you need to do the right thing for people in your care including their families, and so, often, you may be faced with a decision to choose between two or more equally valid options. Good ethical practice requires you to consider the benefits or risks of taking a decision within your field of practice. In other words while the evidence may not have been cut and dried you will need to decide whether to proceed with a change in practice.

Implementing the evidence

Having weighed up the evidence you decide that you want to adopt a particular approach to therapeutic communication within your clinical setting. However, so often in such circumstances good intentions fail because of barriers to the implementation of evidence-based practice. Therefore, careful consideration of the dissemination phase is as crucial to the success of this project as is the literature search and appraisal.

Dissemination strategies

Implementing any new approach to care or treatment involves some degree of change management. In this case it is an anticipated change and effective evidence-based practice requires planning and preparation as well as commitment and motivation from all expected to be involved in the initiative.

Lewin (1951) describes four helpful parameters that should be adhered to when implementing change:

1. Change should only be implemented for good reason
2. Change should be gradual
3. Change should be planned, not sudden
4. All individuals who may be affected should participate in planning for change.

The introduction of therapeutic communication approaches will be the proposed change and is justified by a sound underpinning evidence base. It will involve all affected by the change, including staff colleagues, service users and other members of the team. It will need to be supported by appropriate training and ongoing supervision. It is helpful also to consider some of the common barriers to change in order to plan through how these might be addressed. Resistance due to long-established working practices, attitudinal aspects arising from the perceived threat of change, anxiety provoked by a lack of skills in supporting the change, professional jealousies when change is perceived as encroaching on another's territory and practical aspects such as shift patterns are all commonly encountered. While not easy to overcome, if such barriers are anticipated you are more likely to be prepared and to be able to navigate your way through.

> **Implementing change: a warning**
> The challenge for practitioners is getting approval and commitment for change from colleagues. It requires leadership and the ability to work the change into shifts and work patterns that already exist. Do not underestimate this part of implementation. The research is the first step and has to be seen in this context. It is important to implement change with care and sensitivity. See Chapter 4 for the impact of institutional and group dynamics.

Reflective practice

Any process of change will require the ability to use reflection to learn from and develop practice. It is particularly useful when faced with complex decisions where you are trying to make sense of a situation and move forward. The reflective process will help you tease out influencing factors and determine an appropriate course of action. Much has been written about the value of reflection in and on action and, whatever the theory, it is sufficient to say that reflection helps to appreciate the interrelationship between practice and the environment and to develop insights into one's own influence on the change process. It is through such understanding that you will maximize the potential for success, which in turn will lead to improvements in the standards of care.

> **Case Study 6.1**
>
> *Continued*
>
> Having considered the evidence you decide to implement a therapeutic communication approach for people who are withdrawn and isolated, adopting a model that has proved moderately successful, with adults, conducted in a similar treatment setting. You already have extensive experience of therapeutic communication from which to draw and have engaged other members of the team and service users in discussions, explaining the background to and underpinning evidence for the approach. Everyone is in agreement and you begin to identify suitable potential participants, based on pre-determined criteria.

Conclusions

This chapter has provided a practical example of how to identify clinical questions and to seek out, appraise and implement evidence in practice. The need to adopt such an approach is emphasized by the professional requirement for nurses to use up-to-date knowledge and evidence to assess, plan, deliver and evaluate care, communicate findings, influence change, and promote health and best practice. While empirical sources of knowledge are not the only ones available, and not all clinical questions can be answered by science, evidence-based practice remains an essential tool for the effective nurse who is seeking to deliver care at the forefront of their discipline.

References

Barker P (2009) *Psychiatric and Mental Health Nursing: The Craft of Caring.* London: Hodder Arnold.

Birmingham Critical Appraisal Skills Programme (2011) Online: www.casp-birmingham. org/ (accessed 20 June 2011).

Burnard P (2003) Ordinary chat and therapeutic conversation: phatic communication and mental health nursing. *Journal of Psychiatric and Mental Health Nursing* **10**(6), 678–82.

Care Quality Commission (2011) Online: www.cqc.org.uk/ (accessed 20 June 2011).

Dollaghan C (2004) *Evidence-Based Practice: Myths and Realities. The ASHA Leader.* Online: www.asha.org/publications/leader/2004/040413/f040413a1.htm (accessed 20 June 2011).

Duncan E, Best C, Hagen S (2010) Shared decision making interventions for people with mental health conditions. *Cochrane Database of Systematic Reviews* **1**, CD007297.

Ersser SJ (1997) *Nursing as Therapeutic Activity: An Ethnography.* Aldershot: Avebury.

Freshwater D (2002) *Therapeutic Nursing: Improving Patient Care through Self-Awareness and Reflection.* London: Sage.

Lewin K (1951) *Field Theory in Social Science*. New York, NY: Harper and Row.

Malone D, Marriott S, Newton-Howes G, Simmonds S, Tyrer P (2007) Community mental health teams (CMHTs) for people with severe mental illnesses and disordered personality. *Cochrane Database of Systematic Reviews* **3**, CD000270.

McKenna H (2009) Evidence-based practice in mental health nursing practice, in Barker P (ed.) *Psychiatric and Mental Health Nursing: The Craft of Caring*, 2nd edn. London: Hodder Arnold.

Muir Gray JA (2001) Evidence-based medicine for professionals, in Edwards A, Elwyn G (eds) *Evidence-Based Patient Choice, Inevitable or Impossible?* Oxford: Oxford University Press, pp. 19–33.

National Institute for Health and Clinical Excellence (2011) Online: www.nice.org.uk (accessed 15 June 2011).

NMC (2008) *The Code: Standards of Conduct, Performance and Ethics for Nurses and Midwives*. London: Nursing and Midwifery Council. Online: www.nmc-uk.org/Nurses-and-midwives/The-code/The-code-in-full/ (accessed 28 May 2011).

NMC (2010) *Standards for Pre-Registration Nursing Education*. London: Nursing and Midwifery Council.

Sackett DL, Rosenburg WMC, Muir Gray JA, Haynes R, Richardson WS (1996) Evidence-based medicine: what it is and what it isn't. *British Medical Journal* **312**, 71–2.

Sackett DL, Straus SE, Richardson WS, Rosenberg W, Haynes RB (2000) *Evidence Based Medicine: How to Practice and Teach EBM*, 2nd edn. London: Churchill Livingstone.

Schardt C, Adams MB, Owens T, Keitz S, Fontelo P (2007) Utilization of the PICO framework to improve searching PubMed for clinical questions. *BMC Medical Informatics and Decision Making* **7**, 16.

Solutions for Public Health, Critical Appraisal Skills Programme (2011) Online: www.sph.nhs.uk/what-we-do/public-health-workforce/resources/critical-appraisals-skills-programme (accessed 22 June 2011).

Storey J, Buchanan D (2008) Healthcare governance and organizational barriers to learning from mistakes. *Journal of Health Organization and Management* **22**(6), 642–51.

CHAPTER SEVEN

Helen Eunson, Gwyn Grout, Jane Pritchard and John Carthy

Developing nursing decision-making skills

Learning outcomes

- Be able to critically evaluate decision-making theory
- Be able to analyse and apply decision-making formulae
- Be able to develop confidence and competence in critical decision-making

Introduction

Nothing is more difficult, and therefore more precious,
than to be able to decide.

(Napoleon Bonaparte)

The aim of this chapter is to provide working examples of decision-making that you the reader, whether a student, qualified nurse or educationalist, can use to enhance practice. The reflective exercises aim to develop skills, knowledge and confidence. The examples described are complex in nature to allow you to understand the influencers that are intrinsic to mental health care. Although the scenarios are drawn from real clinical experiences the details within all scenarios are purely for training purposes and service user/patient confidentiality has been maintained throughout.

There is a wealth of literature examining various elements of clinical decision-making with research dating back to the 1970s. As professionals we are required to make a variety of decisions from simplistic to complex and from singular to multiple on a daily basis. Dependent on the issue, the level of risk and the wishes of the service user, we may often want to involve others relevant to the decision being made. These might include the service user, relatives/informal carers, other professionals, advocates and voluntary agencies. While sometimes we make decisions autonomously, decisions also occur within the context of inter-professional teams and across different agency boundaries. Our responsibility in such situations is to encourage effective working, shared decision-making and to ensure that the choices of service users are respected (Nursing and Midwifery Council (NMC) 2010). Recovery-orientated approaches emphasize the importance of including service users in, and facilitating their, decision-making (Shepherd *et al.* 2008). These approaches have already been discussed in Chapter 4 and are also supported by values-based practice addressed in Chapter 3. Their principles and possible applications should be kept in mind throughout this chapter.

The importance of decision-making in nursing has been outlined by the NMC in its Standards for Pre-registration Nursing (NMC 2010), which states that all nurses must:

practise autonomously, compassionately, skilfully and safely, and must maintain dignity and promote health and wellbeing … All nurses must also meet more complex and coexisting needs for people in their own nursing field of practice, in any setting including hospital, community and at home. All practice should be informed by the best available evidence and comply with local and national guidelines. Decision-making must be shared with service users, carers and families and be informed by critical analysis of a full range of possible interventions, including the use of up-to-date technology. All nurses must also understand how behaviour, culture, socioeconomic and other factors, in the care environment and its location, can affect health, illness, health outcomes and public health priorities and take this into account in planning and delivering care.

(p. 26)

This is a complex expectation for any individual and one we must aspire to achieve. Alongside this professional requirement there is a wealth of policies and guidelines stipulating the need for all health care professionals to provide evidence-based clinical practice which helps to maximize service user care, whilst minimizing the perceived risks (see Chapter 6). We must, of course, be mindful not to overload ourselves with information as this can result in our exceeding our cognitive capabilities and thus have a detrimental effect on our decision-making. With positive attitudes towards clinical decision-making, we can learn how to determine what information is relevant and what is not. This is not easy, and is made more difficult as no two situations are ever the same. However, with experience and practice, supported through reflection and supervision, and a genuine desire to achieve the right outcome we can become good decision-makers.

Decision-making theory

There is a wealth of information available relating to decision-making models and the circumstances and setting in which they are best used. For example SWOT (Strengths, Weaknesses, Opportunities and Threats) analysis (Learned *et al.* 1969) may be useful in considering your own development, force field analysis (Lewin 1997) may help to support change and decision trees (Dowding and Thompson 2004) can help a person decide on the best course of action where precision is required and there are several possible courses of action. However, regardless of which model(s) you choose to use there are five basic principles that are consistent within most models even if not explicitly stated:

1. Define the problem/need

   Is the problem/need clear?

2. Define the desired outcome

   Do you have a clear idea of the outcome that you (and others) want?

3. Identify the options

   Have you got all the options? Can you ask anyone else? What are the implications of each option?

4. Weigh up the pros and cons

   What are the positives and negatives of each option?

5. Decide and act

   Plan the execution? How will you implement your plan? Who else needs to be involved?

Further to the process of decision-making, there are additional factors that influence evidence-based decisions. Thompson and Dowding (2002) discuss how 'weight' is distributed to these influences differently depending on the problem/decision that has to be made. Read the list below and reflect on the potential influences and consider what impact they have on the decisions you or others (such as other professionals, managers, carers and service users) have to make:

1. Clinical experience

   How rich have your previous experiences been? What did you learn from them? (While years in practice do not equate equally to level of experience it does have an impact.)

2. Research evidence

   What evidence is available? Do you know how to search and identify robust literature?

3. Service user preference

   Do you give them all the facts so they can make informed choices?
   Do you ask the service user their opinion?
   Do you know when you are ethically allowed to go against a service-user's preference?

4. Available resources

   Is the necessary equipment available?
   Are specialist staff available?
   Are there funds available?

These questions are further discussed below through the use of case scenarios.

Reflective Exercise 7.1

- Consider a health care-related decision that you recently made. Reflect back: how did you identify or define the problem/need you wanted to resolve?
- How did you arrive at your decision?
- How did you, or would you, choose between several options?
- What were the pros and cons?
- Was it a 'good' decision?

So when we look back on our decisions, how do we make them, and how do we know whether the decision we made was a 'good' one? Was yours a good decision, because …

- You made your decision quickly?
- You took the same course of action that you took the last time you were in a similar situation?
- You did what 'felt' right using your intuition?
- You did what others do, or what they recommended?
- You received feedback afterwards that it was the right decision?
- It was the most acceptable option for the patient/service user?
- You followed the policy/guidance/evidence base?
- It was morally the right thing to do?
- You chose the option with the least likelihood of harm?
- You chose the option with the greatest likelihood of benefits?
- There were no adverse consequences?
- There were good consequences?
- You weighed up the pros and cons of several options first?

For any decision to be a logical, rather than a random act, some kind of criteria similar to those shown above must be applied. For example if you were choosing an ice-cream flavour you might have used tastiness as your selection criterion. You chose the ice-cream that appeared after deliberation to be the flavour you would enjoy the most, so you have chosen according to the 'what you feel will bring you the greatest likelihood of benefits', and this has guided your action. Supposing six months later, when you are on a low-fat diet, you are offered a choice of ice-cream by a well-meaning friend. You don't want to refuse the offer for fear of offending your friend, but at the same time you want to minimize the damage caused to your waistline. On this occasion you might make a different choice from before, and go for the flavour with the lowest fat content, thereby choosing the option with the 'least likelihood of harm'. The criterion for choosing must therefore change according to the situation if the 'best' decision is to be made.

The 'best' decision made in a life or death situation might be one that was made quickly, rather than one based on protracted discussion of the pros and cons of the various options. Conversely, a decision with far-reaching consequences where time is not an issue might require much more detailed analysis and consultation. Learning which criteria are the most relevant to the situation in hand is therefore essential to becoming a better and more logical decision-maker.

To make the best decision we sometimes employ a type of shortcut called a 'heuristic' that can save time and help to filter out irrelevant information. For example, if, when you made your decision, you made it based on what you did the previous time, then you used the 'take the last' heuristic (Gigerenzer *et al.* 1999). While this strategy could certainly save time, and might be useful when making simple decisions with minimal consequences, doing what you have always done, or copying what others always do is not a good long-term strategy. Every situation is unique, and it would be unwise to assume that the previous decision, or the decision made by the other person, is right, without properly testing this.

Along similar lines, the 'availability heuristic' (Tversky and Kahneman 1973) helps us to see important patterns among reams of information and data (e.g. headache + light sensitivity + rash = meningitis) and to act in a certain way as a result. Sometimes, however, in other situations this can lead us to jump to conclusions and make wrong decisions if we don't have the time to reason through the situation.

- Think carefully about the last decision that you made in a rush. How did you make this decision? Did you use any kind of shortcut?

We are now going to look at some other influencers on our decision-making and provide an opportunity for reflection on how these might influence your practice and your decision-making. It is well known that nurses commonly use intuition to help guide their decision-making and it has been argued that this is a strategy often associated with expert nurses (Benner and Tanner 1987). This is supported through work by McCutcheon and Pincombe (2001) and also Lyneham *et al.* (2008), who make a distinction between conscious and unconscious forms of intuition, the former being based more firmly on logic and evidence. All cognitive short-cuts are prone to bias, however, as important information can also be filtered out leading to suboptimum decisions. Thompson (1999) and Greenhalgh (2002) have therefore called for a 'middle ground' where nurses 'follow their hunches' but also apply the logic-based principles of evidence-based practice.

- Can you think of a time when you have used intuition to solve a problem? How did it work out? Were you happy with the decision that you made?

Sometimes we are not the person best placed to make a decision. We may not have enough knowledge or experience of a particular subject, and we may therefore wish to consult others by asking their views either before or after we have made the decision. For this strategy to be successful, it is essential that the person giving the advice or feedback is suitably qualified to do so, and that you understand the process that they used to make their decision. No two situations are ever entirely the same and what works well in one situation might be disastrous in another if you do not have a good understanding of how the decision was made.

- Do you know which decisions you would be expected to make in your current job role and which decisions you would need to refer to others? Who would be an appropriate person to refer to? Who would be inappropriate?

Sometimes a decision is not ours or any other professional's to make. People accessing health care services have the right to make their own decisions, even unwise decisions, unless they have been proven to lack the mental capacity to do this (Mental Capacity Act 2005). The diagnosis of a mental illness is not proof that the person lacks mental capacity, nor is their appearance, lifestyle or choices that they make. Sometimes, therefore, the role of the nurse becomes one of supporting people to make their own decisions. This might mean advocating for the person, ensuring that they have enough information, helping them to understand the risks and benefits involved in each option and ensuring that others respect their right to make their own choice. In these circumstances the 'best' decision would be one that the person finds the most acceptable, and that they have chosen for themselves in an informed way.

- Can you think of an example when you have supported someone in making a decision? What was good and bad about the experience? What did you learn?

As seen above, ideas about how we conduct ourselves and how we treat others must be incorporated into our decision-making process. We must, for example, work within our professional codes of conduct and the law at all times. Policies and procedures often guide us in a similar way, as does the evidence base underpinning the work that we do. Rules can help us to make good decisions, and decisions that are consistent with what everyone else is doing. Often, however, we are confronted with a novel situation that is not explained within the policy, or where there is no research or ethical guidance available. At this point, therefore, we need to look at using additional strategies to make good decisions.

- What types of rules, guidance and evidence influence your practice?

Barker (1999) has argued that morals and ethics are at the heart of decision-making and that 'in every ethical arena we are required to commune with our consciences when engaged in decision making. Having checked with our conscience we must live with the consequences' (Barker 1999, p. 205). A good decision, taking this view, would be one that was compatible with a moral and ethical code. Sometimes, however, the 'right' decision is not clear, and there are conflicting values and principles leading to a moral dilemma. In this situation there is no obvious right or wrong answer and options have to be carefully weighed against one another. For example the right to autonomy of a person who is confused might have to be balanced against his or her right to protection from injury. There is, therefore, a degree of weighing up of options to be done. This will be examined in more detail shortly.

- What morals guide you? Are these the same for everyone? Are they the same as beliefs?

Outcomes (both projected and actual) can be a good way of deciding between options and learning from experience. If safety is the prime concern (for example when administering medication) a good decision would be one that is expected to minimize the risk of harm, or which led to no mistakes or harm occurring. In other situations, for example when assisting a service user in choosing the best type of therapeutic intervention for them, maximizing benefits might be more important. You would know, therefore, that it was a good decision if the option chosen was most likely to bring benefit for the individual in their particular circumstances. You may also wish to revisit this once you have read the related concepts in Chapter 9.

- Can you think of a time when a good decision was made by you, or someone you know, that still led to a poor outcome or vice versa? Do you think that this stops it from being a good decision?

Weighing up the pros and cons of various options in an analytical way, on paper if necessary, is a good way of solving complex or important problems where much is at stake. A person's risk of suicide, for example, might be seen as a set of scales with factors on one end that place a person at risk (e.g. suffering from severe depression, living alone, being in chronic pain, having recently made a will) and protective factors at the other end (e.g. having a good support network, having an objection to suicide for religious reasons, having hope) which can be seen as balancing each other out. Judgement about overall risk is therefore the product of an almost mathematical calculation with numerous pieces of information being sought, interpreted and weighted. The 'right' decision (about whether to facilitate day leave from an inpatient unit for this person for example) would be one based on a thorough analysis of the known risks in this situation. Sometimes in spite of our best efforts, however, the eventual outcome isn't the one that we wanted or expected. Good decisions can still occur alongside bad outcomes and bad decisions alongside good outcomes. Even the most thorough and logical of assessments could not possibly take into account every variable of the millions available. To attempt to do so would be immensely time-consuming and ultimately futile. As human beings we do the best that we can; therefore, we try to do what is reasonable in the circumstances, based on the information we have available. As practitioners we are all responsible for ensuring accurate records are maintained (Barker 2009; NMC 2010). This is how the law, our regulatory body and our employer also judge our actions and our decisions.

The following four case studies invite you to explore the process of decision-making. Your exploration can be achieved individually, in group discussion or through role-play. You will notice that while each case study uses different key skills (as discussed above) in decision-making the underlying principles are the same; it is anticipated that this will offer a variety of learning experiences that can be applied regardless of the clinical environment.

Putting theory into practice

Case Study 7.1

Mr Britton is a 78-year-old man who has presented at the local emergency department having taken an overdose. As a member of the crisis team you have been asked to conduct an assessment of risk and to consider the future need for intervention.

Reflective Exercise 7.2

In preparation for your assessment consider the influences in decision-making discussed earlier along with the reflections you have already carried out.

In reflecting on your previous clinical experience, linked with your learning, you note that the nursing role in working with the person who is suicidal is to 'assess for suicidal risk, assess the mental status, promote safety, explore precipitants and promote alternative coping strategies' (Barker 2009, p. 185). You also note that evidence confirms that there are notable differences for consideration when assessing older people who have self-harmed, as opposed to their younger counterparts (Chew-Graham *et al.* 2008; Manthorpe and Iliffe 2005). You therefore decide to refine your assessment to explore those risk factors particularly pertinent in older people. In terms of available resources, you have searched the database to establish that Mr Britton has not had any previous contact with mental health services. You have established that there will be a bed available should Mr Britton require admission.

Assessment

Reflective Exercise 7.3

Drawing on the literature and your experience, consider the questions you would ask Mr Britton in assessment. What assessment tools can you use?

Case Study 7.1

Continued

Mr Britton is lying on a trolley in the emergency department. He is alert and orientated and ready to engage. The medical team have declared him medically fit for discharge. By talking to Mr Britton and reviewing his clinical notes you establish that late last night, having not been able to get off to sleep, he took a combination of his medications and alcohol with the intention of not waking up in the morning. He wrote a brief note to his daughter and went to bed. He woke some time later, feeling very unwell, got frightened and called an ambulance.

Mr Britton was widowed 18 months ago. In recent months he has become increasingly disabled by his arthritis and, occasionally, uses alcohol to augment his analgesia. He talks about his life as meaningless without his wife and without the ability to tend his allotment. In recent months he has lost contact with his gardening friends. In talking about his suicide attempt he states both that he is embarrassed by it and that part of him wishes that it had been successful. He says that he had been feeling down all day as it was the date of the village show. In previous years he had won prizes for his onions.

In terms of mental status Mr Britton reports some changes in his appetite and that his trousers are looser than they used to be. He does not sleep well, and is often woken by pain in his joints. He spends more time than he used to in bed as he finds this more comfortable. He finds it difficult to concentrate and has stopped listening to *The Archers*, a habit he and his wife held for years. He often finds that he wishes for death to come along.

In exploring Mr Britton's immediate plans he assures you that he has no intention of attempting to take his life again, although he does mention that another method may prove more effective. While he would prefer to go home, he thinks that he may ring his daughter, Julia Hitchcock, and arrange to stay with her for a while. He is ambivalent about being admitted to hospital. Mr Britton agrees that it may be useful to talk with someone about how he feels and whether some medication may be helpful.

Decision-making

Reflective Exercise 7.4

Think back to the reflections you carried out and now use the four basic principles discussed earlier to facilitate your decision-making.

In the case of Mr Britton, as with many other clinical decisions, there is no definitive right or wrong decision. In breaking down the process of your decision-making you may have considered the issues explored below.

1. Define the problem/need(s)

On the surface it appears that the problem is related to Mr Britton, his suicidal act and what to do next. One may also consider the need to decide whether or not Mr Britton is clinically depressed and what the future intervention options may be. The latter may be seen as a secondary decision for contemplation once the initial decision, about where he can safely be, has been addressed.

In defining the problem(s), the nurse needs to be mindful that no decision is made in a vacuum. You need to be aware of, and reflect on, influences founded within your own morality, values and experience. Consider whether the way in which you define the problem, and its potential solution(s), are influenced by Mr Britton's age, his social status, his gender, his ethnic background, etc. Does he, or do his actions, bring to mind any experiences from your professional or personal past? Such influences may bring about a desire in you to be over-protective, risk-averse, over-prescriptive or dismissive. You should also be mindful, when defining the problem, of the influence of power within the nurse–patient relationship and also within the current social setting. Max Weber describes power as 'the probability of persons carrying out their will, even when opposed by others' (1922, cited in Marshall 1999, p. 519). Mr Britton and the nurse are in the emergency department, an environment wherein the traditional power of medicine prevails and where organizational drivers can be seen to significantly influence decision-making; for example, for Mr Britton to move through the system within a defined timeframe. In such an environment both the nurse and Mr Britton may be influenced to act as the environment and circumstances dictate rather than in recognition of Mr Britton's right to be empowered to be actively involved in decision-making. The nurse may find him or herself drawn into a paternalistic prescriptive role owing to the professional role in such an environment. In challenging clinical circumstances there may be a tendency to be over-simplistic in defining the problem. Without due analysis of the problem, the rest of the decision-making process will be flawed.

2. Define the desired outcome

The desired outcome for the professional is one that both seeks to minimize the risk of a further suicide attempt and is desirable for Mr Britton. Mr Britton's desired outcome is to be able to go home either directly or following a short stay with his daughter Julia Hitchcock and to recover from his distressed state, for example possible depression.

3. Identify the options

You will have identified that there are three options open for Mr Britton. He can return home, go to his daughter's or be admitted to the local mental health unit. You have identified that, owing to risk assessment, supported by the literature about depression and suicidality in old age (Chew-Graham et al. 2008; Manthorpe and Iliffe 2005), ongoing intervention from specialist mental health services is indicated.

At this stage in the decision-making process you will probably have decided to seek the opinion of others. With Mr Britton's consent, you talk to both his daughter and a professional, someone with more or different experience than you. Having conducted the reflections suggested above, this process will serve to further promote improved objectivity in your decision-making. Talking to Julia Hitchcock will also enable you to formulate a wider perspective on Mr Britton and his potential feelings and desires, as well as on her desire, or ability, to take some responsibility for her father, should he come to stay with her. The conversation will have provided you with more information against which to assess the probability, likelihood and chance of a further suicidal attempt.

4. Weigh up the pros and cons

While you are keen to work with Mr Britton in order to enable him to recover his mental health, your overriding concern is the risk of him further attempting to take his life. Having knowledge of the literature you know that his age, health and social circumstance place him at heightened risk.

It is clear that inpatient admission will minimize risk. It may have become apparent that this is essential, as the risk is too high to consider anything else, especially if Mr Britton and/or his daughter concur. The benefits of admission may include the opportunity for Mr Britton to reflect on his situation and his future potential and desires, while receiving intervention for a potential depressive illness. It would provide the opportunity for 24-hour observation of his mood and his suicidal thoughts, feelings and desires. Conversely admission may serve to confirm Mr Britton's perceptions of uselessness and emphasize his belief that he is a burden.

Going to stay with his daughter may similarly impact negatively on Mr Britton's esteem. Depending on where Julia Hitchcock lives, there may be complications in the development of an ongoing therapeutic relationship with a care coordinator in the community; for example, if she lives in a different geographical area. You also need to consider the effect on the relationship between father and daughter. How long may this temporary arrangement last? You are aware that, if risk allows, Mr Britton would prefer to go home with ongoing intervention from your colleagues in community mental health services. It may be helpful to use a decision frame to list the potential advantages and disadvantages of each option. Ideally this exercise is best carried out with Mr Britton and his daughter (subject to his agreement).

5. Decide and act

Completion of the decision-making process is best achieved in collaboration, not only with the service user and those close to them but also with colleagues. In this case it will necessarily be with those colleagues who will continue to work with Mr Britton following your intervention. In concluding and acting on your clinical decision your next act is to fully record your assessment, conclusions and actions in line with your code of professional conduct and local protocols.

Case Study 7.2

Mrs Guthrie is a 44-year-old woman who was admitted to an inpatient ward suffering from an acute episode of psychosis. You are the primary nurse allocated to be responsible for the nursing care and making recommendations during her forthcoming care programme approach (CPA).

Through your discussions with Mrs Guthrie and her husband, your observations and your review of all clinical notes you establish that she suffers intermittently from acute episodes of psychosis but generally lives a fulfilling life in the community with her husband. Mrs Guthrie has disclosed to you that following a weekend away when both she and her husband indulged in illegal substances (cannabis and cocaine) her mental health has deteriorated – there is a history of relapse following substance misuse. She maintains her anti-psychotic medication and accepts it is helpful with minimal side effects. On further exploration you discover Mrs Guthrie would prefer not to take illegal substances but feels under pressure when she is with her husband as she believes he is always supportive and understanding of her mental health issues and he feels it is his release on only a couple of occasions each year at music festivals. Mrs Guthrie enjoys her job as a sales assistant in a local shop and has a good working relationship with her employer and colleagues. Her employer is aware of previous mental health issues but Mrs Guthrie has never been admitted to hospital before while working for him. She is concerned that her job could be at risk.

During the periods of assessment when you may have used evidence-based assessment tools to determine her mental health, needs and risk you are clear that Mrs Guthrie's mental state is becoming more stable and there are no concerns regarding risks to herself or others. However, she appears to be at risk from substance use and/or her husband's pressure to indulge in drug-taking. Her need to feel a valued part of the community by working is also very important to Mrs Guthrie.

As you did in Case Study 7.1, draw on your knowledge of the literature and experiences to consider the questions you would ask Mrs Guthrie and other professionals. What assessment tools could you use and how will you formulate recommendations? Again this example will explicitly use the five basic principles.

1. Define the problem/need(s)

The initial problem has been to address the psychosis, which can be successfully managed with medication. You may also consider substance misuse to be a significant factor which brought Mrs Guthrie into hospital, how to ensure her employment is not compromised and finally the relationship between Mrs Guthrie and her husband. Already there is clear need to work within a multi-disciplinary team to meet all Mrs Guthrie's needs: a doctor or nurse prescriber to prescribe appropriate medication; a substance misuse practitioner to complete a specialist assessment; a social worker and/ or occupational therapist to liaise regarding employment; and a nurse therapist to undertake family work or offer Mr Guthrie education regarding the impact of illicit substances on his wife's mental state.

As you did for Case Study 7.1, consider what influences will affect your definition of the problem. What have been your experiences in the past? Consider your recovery values and principles – do you actively listen to Mrs Guthrie? Can you accept that she is an expert-by-experience and knows her mental health issues better than any health professional looking in? Did you observe your colleagues listening to Mrs Guthrie? Do different disciplines have different powers or influences?

Once you have identified the problem or need(s) you can start to consider how you will recommend they are addressed through the CPA process.

2. Define the desired outcome

The professionals' desired outcome for Mrs Guthrie is to support her in maintaining mental health wellbeing through managing the conflicting factors in her life, for example support from her husband and substance misuse. Mrs Guthrie's desired outcome is to be able to return home and return to her meaningful employment.

3. Identify the options

There are two main options: Mrs Guthrie can remain in hospital or can be discharged. Discharge could be influenced by what follow-up would be available from the community mental health team (CMHT). It is here your risk assessments will be helpful and using strengths-based assessments can prove useful in working with risk (Morgan 2007). This type of assessment will allow you not only to address Mrs Guthrie's current presentation but also to look to the future and pre-plan. Through jointly agreeing positive risk-taking and the service user's personal safety plan you will achieve collaboration between yourselves (the professionals), Mr Guthrie (carer) and Mrs Guthrie (service user). The wider perspective, as in Case Study 7.1, will allow you to seek others' opinions and understand Mrs Guthrie's situation.

4. Weigh up the pros and cons

There is an option to recommend Mrs Guthrie remains in hospital until her psychosis is relieved. However, recovery is about managing symptoms to lead a meaningful life so you may consider a short admission with intensive follow-up in the community to support her in maintaining her strengths and to be able to return to work – something which offers her a great amount of pleasure. Your medical or nurse prescriber colleagues can review Mrs Guthrie's medication and with her full understanding (consistent with mental health legislation) will be able to ensure she remains happy with any alterations.

Substance misuse specialists who can carry out assessments will be able to offer support particularly in relation to relapse/lapse prevention. Mrs Guthrie has already told you she does not like to take illicit substances but feels under pressure from her husband. This pressure may be real or perceived, and unless you engage Mr Guthrie in this process it may be more difficult to support positive change. Education regarding the impact of substances on mental health may not be understood by Mr Guthrie and as he indulges only twice a year and is supportive to his wife he may just not be aware.

Supporting Mrs Guthrie to return to work will involve balancing the scales and considering the positives of returning against the stress work can cause. Engaging her employer (with Mrs Guthrie's consent) may prove beneficial; however, one must remember the need to maintain confidentiality. This is an opportunity to allow Mrs Guthrie to decide how much, if any, her employer should know. Discussing legal frameworks such as employment law may alleviate Mrs Guthrie's anxieties as well as challenging any negative beliefs with the facts that her employer is, on the whole, supportive.

5. Decide and act

It is time to consider your recommendations and fully document them for the CPA. Listening to Mrs Guthrie is of paramount importance and working collaboratively with colleagues and carers will undoubtedly improve the quality of the actions you recommend.

Reflective Exercise 7.6

- Observe colleagues involved in the CPA process – how are plans agreed with service users and written with a strengths-based focus?
- Do you actively listen to service users?
- Do you feel confident to provide expert nursing recommendations?
- Whom can you ask to support you?

Case Studies 7.1 and 7.2 demonstrated a structured process using five stages: defining need, defining outcome, identifying options, considering the pros and cons, and decision-making. Case Study 7.3 will develop your skills further by helping you to consider more angles in your decision-making, and Case Study 7.4 takes you one step further by introducing critical evaluation in the process. Before you begin, refresh yourself by re-visiting your initial reflections at the beginning of this chapter.

Case Study 7.3

You are working in a community mental health team and are asked to visit a 75-year-old woman, Mrs Brown, at her home. She has been referred to your team by her general practitioner (GP), who feels that she needs to go into a care home as both he and social services are concerned that she can no longer look after herself and is refusing help. They believe that she may have a kind of dementia and are asking you to see her in order that this can be confirmed and a suitable placement found.

When you arrive at Mrs Brown's home you notice that the front garden is very overgrown and the porch door is ajar. Mrs Brown greets you warmly, and invites you into her sitting room, which is stacked high with old newspapers and assorted pieces of clothing. Your initial impressions are that the GP and social worker might be correct in their assertions, but you recognize that you need more information.

Reflective Exercise 7.7

- What are your first thoughts about Mrs Brown?
- Think back to the 'availability heuristic' – what trap could you fall into here unless you obtain more information?
- You have already used visual cues to aid your decision-making. You now use your other senses and notice that the house appears to smell of freshly baked bread (olfactory cue), that you can hear birds singing in the next room (auditory cues) and that the wooden floor feels smooth, rather than sticky, under your feet (tactile cue). The newspapers seem to all be fairly recent and have been carefully stacked into piles (visual cues). Your intuition tells you that Mrs Brown is not confused or unable to care for herself and that there is something else happening here.
- What do these additional cues add to the picture of Mrs Brown that you are beginning to construct?
- What evidence do you have so far that she might have dementia and what evidence is there against this?
- Could there be alternative explanations for the untidiness of the house?

Case Study 7.3

Continued

You ask Mrs Brown some questions about herself, including whether she has any family. She says that she has lived in this house all of her life and has no family since her husband died two years ago. She keeps pet budgies, which are a huge source of companionship to her, and she is able to name each of them and describe their feeding schedule. She has visits from friends regularly and she leaves the porch door open when she knows that they are coming as she does not always hear the doorbell when it rings.

Mrs Brown says that she recently had some help around the home following a knee operation, but that she has now cancelled this as she is feeling much better. Her motivation to cook has not been good of late, and she has had a poor appetite. She does, however, continue to bake her own bread twice a week, although most of this she gives to the wild birds in her garden. You notice that there are several bird feeders on the patio. She says that she has never liked gardening and cannot afford to pay for a gardener.

You enquire about the newspapers that she has been collecting and she says that since her husband died she feels a compulsion to collect these, but she cannot explain why. You look again at the items of clothing placed on the chairs and notice that they are all items of male clothing. You ask her about her husband and whether she feels that she has been able to come to terms with his death. She says that she has not. She makes poor eye contact during your conversation with her, is tearful at times and apologizes frequently for the state of the house. She is not sleeping and her clothes appear a little loose on her. When you carry out cognitive testing you find no evidence of cognitive deficits, and she denies forgetting things or having accidents around the home. When you use a depression screening tool this reveals evidence of low mood. She says that she feels low in mood, but would not harm herself in any way.

You conclude that there is no evidence that Mrs Brown has dementia, and you suspect that her obsessional behaviour (hoarding of items) and depression may be linked to the death of her husband. She requests some ongoing support from the CMHT in helping her to come to terms with his death, which you agree to arrange.

Reflective Exercise 7.8

- Did some of the initial cues make you jump to conclusions?
- What would have been the consequences for Mrs Brown if you had not kept an open mind?
- What have you learned from this experience? You may wish to refer back to Chapter 2 to consider the psychological theories that you might have drawn on in relating to Mrs Brown.
- Will you change anything in your practice as a result?

As you did for Case Study 7.3, consider your previous reflections and the elements within the decision-making process that are important? Do you feel confident to make decisions?

The forcible administration of medication against an individual's will is a breach of a person's autonomy and yet may be justified by health professionals as being in the individual's best interests. Most individuals detained under the Mental Health Act (MHA) 1983, amended 2007 (Department of Health (DH) 2007) can be given treatment for their mental disorder without their consent.

Case Study 7.4

Mr Smith is a 28-year-old man transferred from prison under restriction (MHA 1983, amended 2007 section 47/49) to a high secure hospital. During the past six months, the prison staff had become concerned that Mr Smith was increasingly disengaged and paranoid, he felt prison officers were poisoning his food and he would pace his cell muttering, sometimes shouting. There was no psychiatric history and he had not had contact with psychiatric services previously. He was admitted to hospital for assessment and treatment.

Initially Mr Smith was co-operative and willing to engage with nursing staff and other clinical team members. But it was difficult to elicit information from him about his behaviour in prison and there were no overt symptoms of mental disorder. Nursing staff influenced a decision not to introduce medication at this stage, preferring to develop rapport and increase engagement with him in order to understand his presentation while in prison, which may have been due to illicit drug use or other organic cause.

Within two weeks of admission, Mr Smith was spending extended periods of time in his room, demonstrating irritability with nursing staff, and he seemed increasingly troubled and preoccupied. The clinical team reviewed his presentation and decided that he should be offered psychotropic medication. During the next week nursing and medical staff met with Mr Smith daily to discuss medication options. He declined oral medication but eventually agreed to have an intramuscular psychotropic medication; however, when nursing staff attempted to administer this he became distressed and refused to have the medication. Subsequently he appeared hyper-vigilant and suspicious and refused to discuss medication. His behaviour was causing concern, he was isolating himself, scrutinized all staff about why he was in hospital and refused to talk about his psychological distress.

In the third week after admission Mr Smith was observed to be pacing in his room, constantly muttering and frequently shouting. He was making threats to nursing staff, the junior doctor and other patients to stay away from him. He was angry about staff interfering with his food and was frightened that other patients may attack him. He also indicated that if staff came to administer medication he would

continued ➤

fight them. Mr Smith did not feel he was ill and did not accept he needed treatment in hospital. The clinical team agreed that Mr Smith was demonstrating acute symptoms of paranoid psychosis. He appeared to lack capacity and was not agreeable to taking oral medication. A decision to seek a second opinion was taken. The second opinion approved doctor (SOAD) attended within three days, and, following interviews with Mr Smith and members of the clinical team, the SOAD agreed that intramuscular medication was an appropriate treatment. Given Mr Smith's stated resistance to accepting treatment the nursing team had to prepare to forcibly medicate him against his will.

A discussion about the merits of forcible medication without informing the patient as opposed to providing information to Mr Smith about the team's intentions produced a number of scenarios, each of which were weighed to determine a clinical team consensus. Competing principles, including duty of care, greatest good, autonomy, non-maleficence and justice, were considered. The risk of serious assault may be increased if the team informed Mr Smith, in advance, of their intentions to administer intramuscular medication, thus losing the advantage of surprise designed to reduce the risk of harm to staff. Ultimately his consistent hyper-vigilance meant that he was likely to respond violently whether he was aware or not of the details of the intervention.

Case Study 7.4

Continued

The primary nurse and junior doctor agreed to meet with Mr Smith daily during the next seven days to explain the decision to administer medication by injection, the type of medication to be used, its effect and possible side effects and to attempt to gain his agreement to the procedure. In the meantime consideration had to be given to managing the risk of violence to staff administering the medication. An HCR-20 (Webster *et al.* 1997) violence risk assessment was completed; this comprehensive assessment takes account of historical, clinical and risk factors to provide predictive risk scenarios. Mr Smith had a history of serious assaults on others within the context of suspiciousness; these incidents were preceded by threats to assault and threats to kill. The nursing team in collaboration with (prevention and management of violence and aggression) (PMVA) staff developed plans for restraint and administration of medication.

Following the SOAD interview and during the period the team members were discussing medication with him, Mr Smith was observed to be engaging in physical exercise within his room (press-ups, sit-ups, stretches and shadow-boxing); he was thought to be preparing to violently resist intramuscular medication. Mr Smith was medication naïve and the clinical team gave consideration to the initial dose and side effects, including the possibility of acute side effects. There was also discussion about the risks of inadvertent administration of a long-acting psychotropic medication into a vein as well as the risk of needle-stick injury to nursing staff or Mr Smith if he were to struggle violently during the administration procedure. In preparing for forcible administration the clinical team was cognizant of the guidance provided within the *Code of Practice: Mental Health Act 1983* (DH 2008). This provides a set of guiding principles which should be considered when making decisions about a course of action under the Act. It states:

> *The method chosen must balance the risk to others with the risk to the patient's own health and safety and must be a reasonable, proportionate and justifiable response to the risk posed by the patient.*

> *(DH 2008, p. 117).*

Case Study 7.4

Continued

Two days before the administration of medication the clinical team met with senior managers and PMVA representatives to review plans. Mr Smith's sleep pattern was increasingly poor as were his appetite and personal hygiene.

Concerns were raised about his increasingly violent threats towards anyone who might restrain him or attempt to medicate him; his threats were at times homicidal in nature. Consideration was given to the use of personal protective equipment (PPE) – anti-stab vests, helmets, protective clothing and shields – to reduce the risk of harm to staff involved in his restraint.

The use of protective equipment is strictly controlled by a hospital policy and has to be authorized by an executive officer at the request of a PMVA clinical specialist in collaboration with the clinical team. On this occasion it was felt that a request for authorization did not meet the criteria for PPE use. The team agreed that Mr Smith was suffering a mental disorder, he was acutely distressed and his psycho - social functioning was rapidly declining, at the same time his risk of harm to others was increasing. A final consensus was reached to proceed with forcible treatment to prevent further deterioration.

Reflective Exercise 7.9

The final decision to proceed was the culmination of a number of related, complex decision steps involving nursing staff, the multi-disciplinary team members, senior managers and PMVA staff. With reference to relevant guidelines and evidence, identify and critically evaluate the ethical and legal considerations in the decision steps to forcibly medicate a person in care.

Conclusion: opportunity for reflection

In this chapter we have described the nature and process of decision-making as it constantly occurs within clinical nursing practice. We invited the reader to explore possible decision-making strategies while being mindful of intrinsic and extrinsic influencing factors. It is clear that there is no clear definition of what constitutes a 'good' decision, or a 'bad' decision, as outcomes are never wholly predictable. However, it is clear that the more skilled a clinician becomes, both in their clinical repertoire and in their ability to reflect, the more likely they are to make informed decisions with service users.

In conclusion we invite you to reflect on your learning for the experience of working through this chapter:

- What did you learn from working through the exercises and scenarios?
- Was one more difficult than the others? Why do you think that was?
- Have you witnessed any similar decisions in clinical practice?
- Were the 'right' decisions always made?
- Would you make the same decision on another occasion?
- How do you intend to extend your practice further?

And finally:

In any moment of decision the best thing you can do is the right thing,
the next best thing is the wrong thing,
and the worst thing you can do is nothing.

(Theodore Roosevelt)

References

Barker P (1999) *The Philosophy and Practice of Psychiatric Nursing.* London: Churchill Livingstone.

Barker P (ed.) (2009) *Psychiatric and Mental Health Nursing: The Craft of Caring,* 2nd edn. London: Hodder Arnold.

Benner P, Tanner C (1987) How expert nurses use intuition. *American Journal of Nursing* **87**(1), 23–34.

Chew-Graham C, Baldwin R, Burns A (2008) *Integrated Management of Depression in the Elderly.* Cambridge: Cambridge University Press

DH (2007) *Mental Health Act 1983 as Amended by the Mental Heath Act 2007.* London: TSO.

DH (2008) *Code of Practice: Mental Health Act 1983.* London: TSO.

Dowding D, Thompson C (2004) Using decision trees to aid decision making in nursing. *Nursing Times* **100**(21), 36.

Gigerenzer G, Todd PM, ABC Research Group (1999) *Simple Heuristics That Make Us Smart*. Oxford: Oxford University Press.

Greenhalgh T (2002) Intuition and evidence; uneasy bedfellows? *British Journal of General Practice* **52**, 395–9.

Learned EP, Christiansen C, Roland AK, Guth WD (1969) *Business Policy: Text and Cases*. Scarborough, Canada: RD Irwin.

Lewin K (1997) *Resolving Social Conflicts and Field Theory in Social Science*. Washington, DC: American Psychological Association.

Lyneham J, Parkinson C, Denholm C (2008) Explicating Benner's concept of expert practice; intuition in emergency nursing. *Journal of Advanced Nursing* **64**(4), 380–7.

Manthorpe J, Iliffe S (2005) *Depression in Later Life*. London: Jessica Kingsley.

Marshall G (1999) *Oxford Dictionary of Sociology*. Oxford: Oxford University Press.

McCutcheon H, Pincombe J (2001) Intuition; an important tool in the practice of nursing. *Journal of Advanced Nursing* **35**(3), 342–8.

Mental Capacity Act (2005) *Code of Practice*. London: TSO.

Morgan S (2007) *Working with Risk*: *Practitioner's Manual*. Brighton: Pavilion Publishing.

NMC (2010) *Record Keeping Guidance for Nurses and Midwives 2010*. London: NMC. Online at: www.nmc-uk.org (accessed 16 June 2011).

Shepherd G, Boardman J, Slade M (2008) *Making Recovery a Reality*. London: Sainsbury Centre for Mental Health.

Thompson C (1999) A conceptual treadmill; the need for 'middle ground' in clinical decision making theory in nursing. *Journal of Advanced Nursing* **30**(5), 122–9.

Thompson C, Dowding D (2002) *Clinical Decision Making and Judgement in Nursing*. Edinburgh: Churchill Livingston.

Tversky A, Kahneman D (1973) Availability: a heuristic for judging frequency and probability. *Cognitive Psychology* **5**, 207–32.

Webster CD, Douglas KS, Eaves D, Hart SD (1997) *HCR-20: Assessing Risk for Violence (Version 2)*. Vancouver, BC : Simon Fraser University.

Leading and managing mental health care

Learning objectives

- To develop knowledge of applied nursing leadership and its management and its importance in nursing practice
- Be able to delineate management and leadership tasks
- To develop familiarity with frameworks for leadership and management

Introduction

In this chapter we will consider both the understanding and the development of applied leadership and management skills in mental health nursing. It is relevant to both pre-registration nurses and those post-registration nurses who wish to develop their skills in this key area of nursing practice. It offers examples of leadership and management from a mental health service, illustrating important issues within this essential domain of nursing practice. The mental health service used in the examples is a small psychosis service offering psycho-social interventions for people experiencing psychosis, and for their families. The chapter also offers frequent learning opportunities from mental health practice which can be undertaken individually or within a group to further the understanding of these concepts.

The government's National Health Service (NHS) health care policy is in a continuous state of flux as new evidence of clinically effective treatments emerges, the needs of a population change, and economic or political pressures differ. However, most key NHS documents in the past 10 years or so have consistently emphasized the message that nurse leadership is a powerful influence on clinical standards and should be developed, e.g. *The NHS Plan* (Department of Health (DH) 2000), *Ten Essential Shared Capabilities* (Hope 2004). These policy documents position effective nurse leadership and management at the heart of nurse-led health care delivery in the NHS.

Effective leadership and management in health care settings by nurses are crucial elements in enhancing and maintaining both the quality and the experience of delivered care. Leadership and management determine what care is offered and by whom, and how, when and where care is delivered. Nurses as frontline clinicians are in a position to have an advantaged perspective on the health care needs of their service users, and a working knowledge of care delivery. For mental health care services this knowledge is further advantaged by the therapeutic relationship that exists between the service user and the mental health nurse, allowing for more in-depth information to be gleaned about how care and services can be best organized and delivered. So the very work we, as mental health nurses, do apprentices us for leading and management nursing roles. Becoming a nurse manager or leader requires an organizational-level knowledge of NHS structures and procedures, which is unlikely to be well developed at the beginning of a nursing career. However, there are other more person- and professional-based skills that can be developed and that underpin the wider skills of nurse leadership and management.

We will begin by briefly defining the terms leadership and management and positioning them in the nursing profession; these functions will then be explored in detail throughout the chapter. The chapter will conclude with a description of a developmental journey for leadership and management competency.

> ### Reflective Exercise 8.1
>
> Take a moment to identify a 'leader' from any sphere of life that you admire. What are the qualities that you like about that person?

Leadership and nursing

I am an encourager and a persuader and an advocate.

(*John Howard, Australian Prime Minister, 1996–2007*)

Leadership can be defined as going first and guiding the way for others. It implies having a vision of an objective, a sense of how to attain that objective, and a method of bringing others with you to achieve that objective as an agreed goal. In nursing terms, clinical leadership means taking the leading role in guiding others towards adopting a particular clinically focused behaviour. Anything can be led: clinical care, governance procedures, team culture and implementation of guidelines or policies. Leading is a continuous part of the nursing role and all mental health nurses have a responsibility to contribute to leadership, management and service development (Nursing and Midwifery Council (NMC) 2010).

Leadership strategies are important in facilitating optimum standards in the practice environment (Henderson and Winch 2008); indeed, effective nurse leadership is central to the success of *The NHS Plan* (DH 2000; Mullally 2001). As long ago as 1994, the United Kingdom Central Council for Nursing, Midwifery and Health Visiting (UKCC), now the NMC, stated that nurse leaders were expected to epitomize advanced nursing practice through:

> *adjusting the boundaries for the development of future practice, pioneering and developing new roles responsive to changing needs ... advancing clinical practice, research and education to enrich professional practice as a whole.*

Understanding leadership could be argued to be central to the goals of the nursing profession. While the literature is unclear on the concept of nurse leadership, the varying definitions include the qualities of clinical expertise, inter-personal and communication skills, and empowering staff (Harper 1995). Interestingly, it does not follow that nurse leaders have to be in a senior or managerial position within the organization, nor that clinical leaders have to have a 'vision' of best practice (Stanley 2008). Stanley suggested that it was more 'how' the leader translated their values and beliefs into observable practice and the peer admiration that followed.

Reflective Exercise 8.2

Reflect on a nurse leader you admire. What values were explicit or implicit in their approach to leadership?

The Royal College of Nursing (RCN) noted in 2003 that an integral part of nursing was a responsibility to lead care, lead other nurses and, themselves, to participate in being led by others. While emphasizing leadership, this statement also highlights an aspect of leadership which is often overlooked and that is the art of following, or followership as it is now becoming known. The term 'follower' can be viewed as a pejorative term, as a passive and less valuable role; this is absolutely not so. The roles of leader, manager and follower work most effectively in partnership and are reciprocal; one cannot lead without followers or follow without a leader, and how could we manage effectively if we had no one allowing themselves to be managed? Leaders and managers have rights commensurate with their role but equally have an inherent responsibility to and for their followers. In the same way, followers have rights, but they too have responsibilities towards their managers or leaders. While some of us may not choose to be a leader or a manager during our professional careers, all of us will be a follower.

> **Reflective Exercise 8.3**
>
> What skills and attributes make a good 'follower'? Is leading more important than following?

The art of followership includes such skills as:

- A willingness to accept guidance and direction from leaders and managers
- Taking responsibility for one's own actions
- Supporting the leader in their leadership tasks
- Questioning the rationale for requested actions
- Advocating for the rights of the receivers of such actions, i.e. service users.

An effective follower needs to be flexible and co-operative, open to both instruction and potential criticism from their leader without becoming defensive or challenging. Equally, followers have a responsibility to develop an assertive style of seeking clarity for the rationale underpinning a leader's directions. Following should never be a 'blind' role and effective leaders will empower followers to be active and collaborative. See also Chapters 2, 3 and 4 of this book for issues regarding self-awareness in relation to roles within the family or a group as leader or follower.

> **Reflective Exercise 8.4**
>
> Reflect on a nursing practice experience where you were a follower. What followership skills did you utilize that helped you be an effective follower to another's lead?

Management and nursing

Surround yourself with the best people you can find, delegate authority, and don't interfere.

(Ronald Reagan, President of the United States of America, 1981–99)

Management happens in every domain of life, from self-management to corporate management. The term 'management' can be sourced to both Latin and French, and is defined as 'to conduct or direct'. It could be argued that to manage is to effectively utilize and co-ordinate resources to meet defined objectives. It is a definition that does not lend itself easily to our caring profession, but without nursing management it is unlikely that nursing could operate effectively, professionally or safely. A more acceptable definition might be that nurse management is a continuous process of planning, leading, organizing and evaluating a team of people in order to achieve both required and agreed goals and standards, and doing so within resource limits. A wordy definition indeed, and yet effective management is still easier to define than to accomplish!

Health care or nurse management has the additional dimension to most managed arenas as it deals with vulnerable people and is often forced to make decisions and choices which allocate resources or make a decision in favour of one health care need against another. Moreover, the actual and ethical ramifications of substandard care or unprofessional behaviour have an increased seriousness because they impact detrimentally on people who are vulnerable.

Wiggins and Hyrkäs (2011) suggest that there are several evidence-based management practices for health care management, and effective management is the skill in translating such evidence-based approaches into practice. These practices include: balancing tensions between productivity and efficiency; actively managing the process of change; and sustaining trust. All of these are highly relevant to the ebb and flow of NHS policy and ensuing reorganization of resources. Nurse management, then, encompasses a myriad of tasks and responsibilities directed at ensuring the optimum operation of a service, within parameters ascribed by the wider organization and professional bodies, and within finite resources, to ensure optimum standards of care are delivered.

Are management and leadership exclusive functions?

Management is doing things right; leadership is doing the right things.

(Peter Drucker, writer, 1909–2005)

Leadership is currently fashionable and management often denigrated, but both are important and need to work concurrently. It is through management and leadership that the quality and experience of care is maintained and enhanced. Is it useful to separate leadership and management? Can you lead outside of a management role, can you manage without leading? Whitehead *et al.* (2007) suggest that it is the combination of three qualities which make an effective manager: leadership, clinical expertise and business sense. Pullen (2003) describes leadership skills as including self-knowledge, communication skills, risk-taking and keeping informed. Combining the two skillsets, we can see that operating as an effective nurse manager is a highly skilled role, but not one that is separate from leadership; indeed leadership is an integral element of management. This would suggest that you cannot be an effective manager without leadership knowledge and skills; and you cannot be an effective leader without management knowledge and skills. However, it does not imply that you have to be a manager to lead or a leader to manage; some managers will chose leads within their team to fulfil a variety of leadership functions and utilize their own management skills to create a balanced team, and equally some leaders will delegate management functions to team members to create balance.

Each nurse will have a natural inclination towards leadership or management, and it is the recognition of your own skillset and consideration of how to utilize this appropriately in a nursing role that will develop effective leading and managing competency. However, it is interesting to note that while every nurse should be a leader, perhaps not every nurse should be a manager (Whitehead *et al.* 2007).

When leadership and management functions are both part of a nurse's role, it is not always easy to know when to lead and when to manage. Doing both functions can cause confusion and frustration, yet both play an important part in supporting the service or team to maintain and enhance standards of care delivery and professional behaviour.

Table 8.1 Delineating managerial and leadership responsibilities

Management responsibilities	Leadership responsibilities
Day-to-day team management and individual practitioner management	Creating a culture of clinical excellence
Referral and caseload management	Staying abreast of best practice in psychosis
Awareness of, adjusting to and monitoring of national, NHS Trust and area operational requirements	Maintaining a high level of knowledge and understanding of the experience of psychosis
Data gathering for NHS Trust performance targets	Developing clinical interventions in line with the most up-to-date evidence base
Allocating resources	Maintaining high standards of own practice
Budget management	Explicitly modelling best practice
Service governance – creating the framework and ensuring team adherence	Maintaining a standard of clinical excellence within the team
Monitoring adherence to NHS Trust policies	Refining the clinical governance framework to maintain and develop optimum clinical practice
Ensuring adherence to NHS Trust strategic decisions	Monitoring clinical practice standards
Ensuring registrations with professional bodies are in order	Accountable for clinical practice of team members
Ensuring professional codes of practice are adhered to	Clinical mentoring of team members
Monitoring work safety of team members	Working in collaboration and partnership with service users to facilitate meaningful interventions and projects
Responsibility for the appraisal process for team members	Developing new service projects in partnership with other area mental health teams
Managing complaints from service users	Clinical supervision of qualified team members and trainees
Ensuring the smooth operation of the team	Guiding clinical development of team members
Creating and sustaining a positive, supportive and healthy team culture	Promotion of the service
Monitoring NHS Trust targets and service agreed objectives	Active involvement in clinical research
Being accountable for the operation of the service	

Table 8.1 represents an attempt to delineate management and leadership functions of the lead clinician role within a psychosis service.

Let us consider the language used to describe the tasks: management tasks utilize verbs such as ensuring, monitoring and adhering. The tasks appear to be about maintaining professional and clinical standards and working in line with defined policies and objectives. There is a co-ordination and allocation function for referrals and resources, and an accountability for the service. The leadership tasks use language such as best practice, clinical excellence and clinical developments. The focus of the management role is inwards towards the team and the lead's focus is outwards, beyond the team. However, both function to ensure the optimum operation of the team in terms of professional behaviour, clinical standards of care and service imperatives.

Reflective Exercise 8.5

Reflect on the delineated tasks in Table 8.1.

- Do you think the tasks should be delineated as shown?
- Are there identified management tasks that you would place in the leader column, and vice versa?
- As a nurse manager, which management or leadership tasks would you delegate to a team member, and how would you support this delegation?
- What would you need in order to feel comfortable with being accountable for a task you had delegated to another person?

Nurse management

This section serves as an introduction to management approaches to set the scene for increasing knowledge and for skill development. There are many fine texts that you can read to build on this knowledge, and one such is noted in the further reading section at the end of the chapter. The nurse manager's role will be a recognized formal appointment by the organization and so have an authority position in the service hierarchy. A nurse manager's responsibilities include:

- Recruitment
- Performance management of staff
- Allocation of finite resources
- Responsibility for ensuring professional standards of care and that behaviours are maintained and improved where appropriate
- Responsibility for ensuring operational fidelity to organizational policy, national guidelines, professional codes and legal statutes

- Being the ultimate decision-maker for the service or team
- Defining the culture of the team; in addition, the nurse manager is accountable for the performance of that team and the individual nurses within the team, in all areas.

The nurse manager role can be an isolative and burdensome one, and propagating support for the management function within the team or service becomes a necessary task. One method of reducing the burden of a management role is to develop from the team a supporting framework of team members to whom management tasks are delegated. Management of the team, its operation and personnel becomes then a shared task and this relieves the strain on the manager. The manager requires confidence in his or her team in order to do this role-sharing as the manager remains ultimately responsible for the actions and decisions of others.

The extent to which a nurse manager leads varies depending on the needs of the service and the skills of the manager. It is important for the nurse manager to recognize his or her own skillset and create roles within the team which support and complement them. In some services there may be separate clinical lead posts; in other organizational structures there will be specified leadership and management responsibilities within the more senior nursing roles. Such tasks within these roles will be a key part of the framework of delegated management and leadership functions supporting the nurse manager role.

So the nurse manager's role is a complex and responsible one, and it is more than the list of tasks, it encompasses the process of 'managing' and this is based on the experience, knowledge and wider skills of the nurse manager. These wider skills will include an understanding of the organizational structures and processes of the service and wider NHS environment, knowledge of the individual team members, service users, the team culture, and the manager's own communication skills and leadership style. A nurse manager needs to know not only the service objectives but also individual team members' objectives. A good manager needs to be well informed about drivers for objectives, as well as have a clear idea of the available resources and capacity of their service to best meet them. In order for these to be effectively managed many factors have to be aligned and considered; Box 8.1 notes some of the tasks and processes undertaken by a nurse manager.

Box 8.1

Summary: nurse management processes and tasks

- Facilitating team members to develop in their mental health nursing role
- Ensuring high quality of the care delivered
- Ensuring care is delivered within service, organizational and governmental guidelines and policies

- Ensuring service and organizational targets are met
- The allocation of finite resources to facilitate necessary care provision
- Monitoring adherence to integrated governance frameworks
- Sanctioning team members within performance management policies
- Recruitment
- Facilitating of communication from lower down in the organizational structure to higher levels
- Managing dissatisfaction among service users
- Managing dissatisfaction among team members
- Prioritizing tasks within the team
- Juggling competing service demands
- Disseminating information to the team
- Facilitating service development in line with organizational parameters and policy
- Negotiation with support teams such as administrative services
- Representing the service at organizational level
- Representing the service at interagency forums

The skills and processes of the nurse management role can be categorized (e.g. Whitehead *et al.* 2007). In this chapter the following categories are used:

- Monitoring
- Decisional
- Relational
- Developmental.

Each category is considered in more detail below and two categories, decisional and monitoring, will consider a management style or approach which might be adopted for that process.

Areas of responsibility in a nurse manager role

Monitoring

The nurse manager role has a high proportion of monitoring responsibilities including:

- The activity of the team or service against specified organizational targets, particularly in terms of clinical activity, governance policies and outcomes
- The professional behaviour of individual team members and their adherence to professional codes of practice and to service and organizational policies, resource use, including the service budget, and allocation of referrals.

The nurse manager will have a personal style of monitoring depending on the task itself, their own values base and their beliefs about the team. A transactional model of management might be used. Transactional management is also known as transactional leadership (Bass 1985). Transactional leadership is an explicit rule-driven form of management, whereby people can be 'rewarded' for adhering to the rules of prescribed behaviour and sanctioned for non-adherence. It can be an informal or formal arrangement where behavioural expectations are explicit and meeting these expectations is recognized in some way. A transactional approach is useful when team members are inexperienced or when there is little time to spend on the idiosyncratic behaviours of team members, and adherence to policies or standards of behaviour is crucial. In terms of monitoring tasks, it is a potentially useful management style as it predicts that team members know what is expected of them and know what they can expect if they do not adhere to such rules. There are disadvantages to this style of management, including creating a dependent team culture, reliant on edicts from management.

Reflective Exercise 8.6

What are your thoughts about being responsible for the monitoring of others' behaviours?

Decisional

The nurse manager is the ultimate decision-maker for the service, whether this is at a service user, individual team member or team level. They are also responsible for implementing organizational decisions. In management and organizational terms, the descriptors 'top-down' and 'bottom-up' indicate the direction of decision-making, objective setting, resource allocation and accountability. For decisional activities this framework can be exceptionally useful to consider how decisions have been informed and the impact they might have. In a top-down model, decisions are made in the higher management structures of the organization, usually by a small group of high-level managers, and these decisions are communicated, or cascaded, down through the organizational layers through the managerial pathway. These traditional management frameworks tend to put the service user at the bottom of the organizational pathway. Service managers then have the task of actioning the decisions in their teams with little autonomy.

A top-down model can be effective though, particularly in large organizations, and in health care it can benefit attempts to standardize service delivery in terms of both quality and availability. There is also a supportive line of accountability: if something is not quite right at the lower end of the organizational hierarchy then responsibility for this can be passed back up the chain. However, criticisms of this decisional framework include the awareness of increased distance between the decision-makers and the service users. This can cause services to fail to reflect the needs of the service users and remove opportunities for service user dialogue to inform service development. Moreover, mangers at service level have to 'impose' decisions on their services and this top-down imposition can make it difficult for decisions to be supported at the lower levels.

In contrast, a bottom-up approach is one that works from the lower levels of the organization – again it places service users at the bottom, but works from them as a primary source of decisional information. This approach allows individuals at the bottom of the organization's framework to identify goals for the organization, and they are likely to better reflect the needs of this organizational level. However, there are disadvantages to bottom-up decisional activity, whether for service users or for employees, in that such decisions may not reflect the organization's responsibilities and many lead to an ad hoc approach to care. An obvious compromise is integrated decisional activities, which takes into equal account the rights and responsibilities of all those involved, but it can be a lengthy process.

> **Reflective Exercise 8.7**
>
> - What are your thoughts about being a decision-maker?
> - What elements of this task arouse concerns for you?

Relational

The relational aspect of nurse management includes the inter-personal arena within which effective management takes place, whether this be supporting a team member through a time of personal difficulty, managing a complaint from a dissatisfied service user, disseminating information or actioning decisions. A nurse manager needs to be able to:

- Communicate effectively with the team and the service users, and disseminate information appropriately
- Communicate through organizational structures as a representative and advocate of the service and its users
- Communicate with agencies external to the service and the organization that have a stake in the functioning of the service, e.g. social services, charitable organizations.

Developmental

The nurse manager is responsible for the consideration of service development and the management of service change to facilitate the meeting of organization targets, demands from its service users, and the supporting of its staff in their ability to operate effectively. And this has to be done within the finite resources available to the service and often to a timescale. This developmental process may be driven by a transformational approach (Burns 1978) or a transactional approach (Bass 1985); it may be democratic or autocratic. It may be a task that the nurse manager delegates to a team member and asks them to lead on it; this may be particularly true if the manager identifies a team member who has attributes of leadership and is an effective management strategy.

Effective nurse management can run a line between micro-management and absentee management. These are two extremes whereby either the nurse manager perceives it necessary to oversee every single team action and decision, or they become distanced from the team and issue edicts from an inaccessible position. Neither of these positions is an optimum mode of management but might develop when a nurse manager feels overwhelmed by management tasks and prioritizes their accountability role, consequently behaving to control the operational and personnel minutiae – in a sense, underestimating the competence of their team. Alternatively, a nurse manager may overestimate the competence or capacity of their team and manage from afar, informing the team of decisions and prescribing behaviours without accepting accountability for the team's functioning or wellbeing.

Mental health nurse management domains

As illustrated in Figure 8.1, being an effective nurse manager could be seen as needing to be fully cognizant of five domains:

- Service users and carers
- Individual team members
- The service as a whole
- External agencies
- The organization within which the service exists.

Reflective Exercise 8.8

Think about a mental health practice environment you are familiar with. Reflect on the role of the nurse manager and identify specific examples of nursing management in action. Pick one example and deconstruct it into the four elements of: monitoring, decisional, communication and developmental.

- What skills and styles did you observe the nurse manager was using?
- Thinking about the responsibilities and accountability that the nurse manager has, can you explain the response, process and outcome of the specified event?
- Can you think of alternative ways of approaching the identified issue from a manager's perspective?

Figure 8.1 illustrates the interplay between these five domains. In fulfilling any of the functions of the nurse manager role an awareness of the impact any decision or action may have in these five domains is required. What can seem to be a simple action within one domain can sometimes have an unforeseen consequence in another. A more

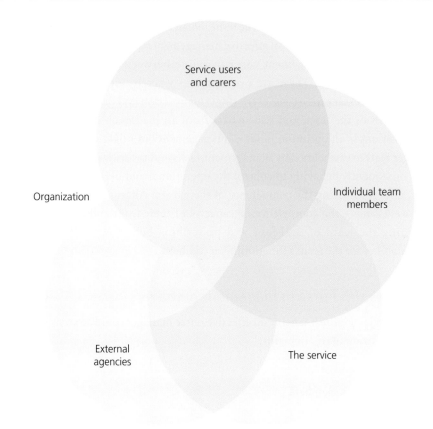

Figure 8.1 The five domains of nurse management.

systemic approach to management pays dividends in predicting impact on other domains and timely action to minimize problems. Juggling the competing demands of domains can be challenging as one domain's demands will often require something from another domain, and this may be resisted or difficult to give from within domains. Whilst the nurse management function can sometimes be a negotiated compromise across domains, it sometimes has to be the imposition of a course of action which may not be popular with one or more of the four domains, and the nurse manager is the person who has to facilitate the choice of solution and manage the potential 'fall out' from the application of such decisions.

Reflective Exercise 8.9

Refer back to Figure 8.1 and reflect on which domain the tasks identified fall into.

Managing competing demands

An emergent evidence base suggests that psychological therapy as an intervention for people experiencing psychosis is more effective when undertaken by a specialist practitioner separately but in conjunction with ongoing active care co-ordination (Brooker and Brabban 2004).

Case Study 8.1

Managing competing demands

Let us assume that a specialist psychosis service, informed by the evidence base, requires that a referral is accepted only if there is an active care co-ordinator. The evidence for the efficacy of adjunctive psychological therapy/care co-ordination is in competition with the referring team's need to manage its own service demands and resources.

The management dilemma includes these issues:

- There is an understandable belief by referrers to the psychosis service that the specialist practitioner has the skillset to manage all of the service user's difficulties rather than only provide the psychological therapy component.

- Referring to the psychosis service does not reduce case loads for the referring community mental health team, which, if it did, would enable service users on the referring service's waiting list to be accepted.

- If a referral is not made to the psychosis service then the service user may not be able to access effective psychological therapy and have a different quality of recovery.

- If the service user is not referred to the psychosis service then recommendations from National Institute for Health and Clinical Excellence (NICE) guidelines may not be adhered to and organizational targets are less likely to be met.

- If the psychosis service accepts a referral without an active care co-ordinator, then the effectiveness of the psychological therapy may be reduced and the quality of care experienced by the service user may be compromised.

Reflective Exercise 8.10

Refer to Figure 8.1 and consider the issues arising for each domain.

Reflecting on these competing demands, how might you manage this situation?

- Is there a range of solutions?
- How do you decide which to choose?
- What nurse management and leadership skills might you utilize to resolve this issue?

Remember that, while you have to attend to all domains, it is best practice to position the service user at the heart of your discussions.

Nurse leadership

Leaders need to be optimists. Their vision is beyond the present.

(Rudy Giuliani, Mayor of New York, 1994–2001)

Leaders do not have to be in a senior or managerial position within the organization, nor do leaders have to have a 'vision' of best practice, it is more that leaders explicitly translate their values and knowledge into observable behaviours and so encourage others to follow their lead (Stanley 2006, 2008). Literature tells us that that the qualities of confidence, competence and self-awareness are necessary for effective leadership, and that accompanying a political awareness and effective teamworking skills is an explicit service user focus (Adair 2002; Alimo-Metcalfe 2003). Leadership is possible in many arenas, from self-leadership to leading individualized episodes of care, from leading a clinical area to team leadership and ultimately to leading service development or wider developments. These domains are interconnected. Figure 8.2 illustrates the domains of leadership, showing the widening of your sphere of influence from self-leadership to

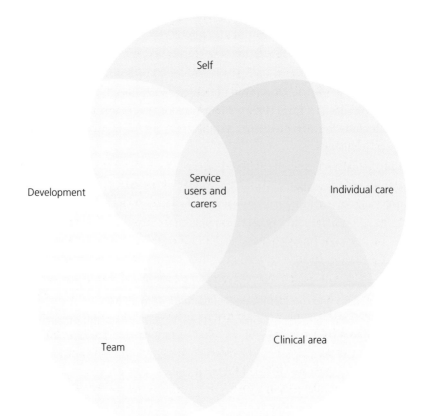

Figure 8.2 The five domains of nurse leadership.

developmental leadership, but always keeping the service user at the heart of leadership actions. Leading in any one domain will influence another. Leading yourself professionally as a mental health nurse will influence the individualized care you lead, while leading a specific clinical area of care will influence wider service development. This is, in turn, influenced by your leadership of your self and the individualized care episodes you have led. These domains reflect the developmental skill acquisition journey described later in this chapter.

The skills needed to be an effective leader include (Pullen 2003; Stanley 2008):

- Approachability and accessibility
- Awareness of own values and the embodiment of these values within actions
- Being an effective communicator
- Being a positive role model
- Being empowered and in a position to make decisions
- Being clinically competent and well informed.

There are a number of leadership theories, of which one, transformational leadership (Burns 1978), has gained popularity in the health care profession in recent years, although it is not without its critics (Stanley 2008). Transformational leaders can achieve higher levels of organizational performance and, in nursing, contribute to improving the quality of care and patient care satisfaction (Marchionni and Ritchie 2008). Transformational leadership involves emotions, motives and ethics and incorporates visionary leadership (Northouse 2004). Transformational leadership qualities include setting direction, establishing a vision, developing people and building relationships.

A transformational leader will first define a vision, this vision being informed by a consideration of the sought and expressed voice of the service user, the literature and evidence base for the 'vision', knowledge of the team resources and culture, and knowledge of political and organizational objectives and guidelines. The use of the term vision does not imply that the leader's objective has to be far-reaching; smaller visions, if well thought through and executed, can be just as important to the service user or the team. Once the vision is defined and informed, a transformational leader will raise the profile of the task with the key stakeholders for the vision; this could be the service users, the team members or other organizational figures. The goal of the transformational leader is to bring people to the idea, and guide them along as an active part of working towards the vision. A transformational leader needs to have reputation and a 'charisma' defined through clinical competency and trust. They are often extemporary role models who are respected by others. They have an ability to motivate and innovate.

Transformational leadership is not always appropriate. It operates most successfully in teams where there is a high level of skill or experience, and less so where teams feel under-confident or stretched, or where there is less opportunity to access everyone's input. In times of short-term crisis, transformational leadership can exacerbate rather than assuage; then a more transactional management and leadership style is appropriate. However, it is highly effective when a team decision-making culture exists, and there is scope for facilitating personal and professional development. With highly skilled or experienced staff, and for visions or changes which can be undertaken at a considered pace, transformational leadership wins through (see also Box 8.2).

Box 8.2

Clinical governance through agreement

An essential function of clinical leadership is the clinical governance of a service or team. Governance operates through procedures put in place to monitor and maintain optimum standards of professional care delivery. Such procedures create a governance framework through which all essential elements of professional care delivery can be monitored and so standards maintained and targets met. They might include adherence to all NHS Trust policies, an operational policy for the service which defines how the service will function and its organizational position, systems for note-keeping and sharing of appropriate information with other involved professionals, evidence-based interventions to be used, adherence to best practice or clinical guidelines such as the NICE guidelines, or clinical or cost targets required to be met.

The psychosis service's clinical governance happens through a framework of clinical processes and procedures which help to maintain and to enhance its clinical delivery. These governance procedures are developed and agreed on by the psychosis team and recorded in a shared document which is reviewed by the team when organizational or policy change occurs, when best practice information changes, or when it is felt by team members or service users that the structures or processes of the service need redefining.

The leader's role is to facilitate the team to be able to fully involve themselves in such important decision-making processes and governance development.

Reflective Exercise 8.11

- What does the leader have to develop within the team for such a democratic process to operate?
- What personal and leadership skills does the lead need to support this team development and facilitate this aspect of the service to continue operating within this model?
- What are the advantages and disadvantages of a transformational leadership approach?

A journey of competency development in nurse leadership and management

There are difficulties in learning leadership and management skills while in the pre-registration role: one such is the student position on the developmental learning pathway of knowledge, understanding and skills which are necessary for effective leadership; another is the position all students by definition have in a team hierarchy and the appropriateness of undertaking leadership or management tasks in that learning role. Understandably, as training progresses the opportunities for developing leadership, if not management, skills increase, but it can feel a difficult area to step into even following registration. The NMC *Standards of Competencies for Pre-registration Nurses* (2010) have a specific domain for nurse leadership and management skills which, as a generic competence, requires that pre-registration nurses must show a potential for continuing development of these skills beyond registration. Specifically for pre-registration mental health nurses, the NMC notes that all mental health nurses must contribute to leadership, management and design of services. The NMC views nurses as agents of change, providing leadership through the route of care and service development to enhance the quality and experience of care. For mental health nurses clinical supervision and reflection are key skills, as is an awareness of personal values and an understanding of how they translate into practice. There is also an expectation of wider promotion of best practice in mental health care.

Reflective Exercise 8.12

Imagine yourself in the role of mentor to a pre-registration student nurse. What learning experience task could you support your student in undertaking that would illustrate how to promote an element of best practice within the clinical placement environment?

Stepping into a more demanding nurse leadership or management role will occur naturally as one progresses through a mental health nursing career, but this would imply that opportunities to develop these skills are not available until expected in a more senior post. Stepping up to more senior and demanding roles and feeling unskilled can be daunting. For nurses moving through their pre-registration training and for those registered nurses who wish to develop their skills in leadership and management, there are ways to approach skill acquisition from pre-registration onwards. It would not be unreasonable for pre-registration nurses to assume that leadership and management is a skillset not easily developed at the starting point of their professional career; however, Figure 8.3, which is based on the NMC (2010) competencies, offers a useful framework for all nurses who wish to develop leadership and management skills even from the earliest point.

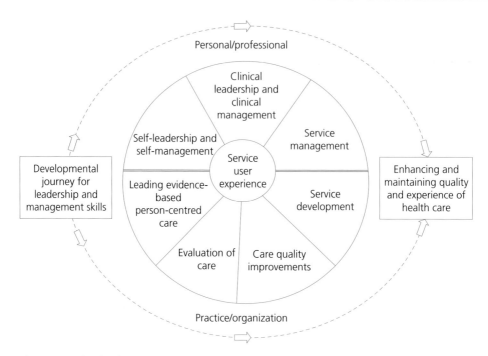

Figure 8.3 The developmental journey of competency.

Figure 8.3 illustrates the journey of competency development. It defines the rationale for development of these nurse management and leadership skills as operating to enhance and maintain the quality and experience of care. This diagram is a useful framework from which to consider your own professional journey of management and leadership development. We all start from the left-hand side of the framework, and, as our knowledge, skills and experience increase (as we spend more time nursing), we can develop personal and professional competencies, moving from self-leadership and management to clinical leadership and management and ultimately to service leadership and management, if we choose to. At the same time, we will have the opportunity to develop our leadership and management skills in the practice and organizational domain by leading a single episode of care to evaluating care provided by ourselves and our colleagues, through to leading care quality improvement and ultimately clinical service development.

Reflective Exercise 8.13

Consider where you are on this framework at the moment; where would you like to be when you consider your professional future?

As shown in Figure 8.3, the learning journey is divided into two domains, the personal and professional, and the practice and organizational. It clearly places the service user experience at the heart of this developmental journey. This emphasizes that, at all stages of competency development, consideration of the needs and rights of the service user are a necessary part of that competency, whether it is through reflecting on why you are entering the field of mental health nursing and how your own values and beliefs influence your interactions with service users, or whether it is collaborating with service users as part of a service development project. Without service users there is no role for mental health nurses!

In the personal and professional hemisphere, competency has been segmented into self-management and self-leadership, clinical leadership and management, and service management with an implicit leadership function.

In the lower hemisphere, practice and organizational, the developmental journey of skill attainment flows from leading individualized care episodes and evaluation of that care through to informing care quality improvements and service developments. To be an effective nurse manager and leader all segments to the left of your current segment of functioning need to be active in your practice. If you are in a clinical lead role, you need to underpin this by effective self-leadership and self-management; to be leading or managing care quality improvements you need to support your efficacy by leading and evaluating individualized care episodes. Remember you can stop at any 'segment' in your mental health nursing career in terms of leadership and management but there is a professional expectation that you will be effective at self-management and self-leadership, and you will certainly be expected to be taking the lead on individual care and evaluating its clinical effectiveness.

Self-leadership and self-management can be viewed as the starting point of the leadership and management skills developmental journey within the personal and professional domain. Self-leadership and self-management are areas of skill attainment open to all mental health nurses from day 1 of their pre-registration course, but also are a first stage for any nurse, mental health or other specialty, wishing to begin their leadership and management skill developmental journey.

Self-leadership and self-management skills cover vast ground and include many issues that could be consider trivial, but are they? Small things such as your appearance, attitude to being at work and being led, and respect and compassion for service users do matter. It is through these initial steps of self-management and self-leadership that your mental health nurse role becomes defined. If we refer back to Figures 8.1 and 8.2, which define the domains across which leadership and management operate, we can begin to build a picture of what self-leadership and self-management include. What might you need to manage about yourself as a mental health nurse when you are interacting with service users and carers? You would need to manage your personal and professional qualities, responsibilities and skills. As a mental health nurse in the community, visiting people in their own homes requires you to manage yourself professionally and remain respectful to the service user. You will need to manage the care you provide, its evaluation and recording. You need to be accessible and reliable. Similarly when working as part of a team you have to manage yourself within that team or as part of a wider service, the organization and your profession. These self-management skills run from the basic requirements of reliability and attitude to more professional issues of effective communication, risk management and clinical skills. And while the former can seem to be stating the obvious, sometimes the obvious is worth stating!

Self-leadership is a very important area as this begins your competency development and needs to be considered within the five domains of Figure 8.2, and in terms of what self-leadership means for the service user. Self-leadership includes motivating yourself to become well informed, politically aware and to lead by example – even pre-registration nurses can be role models of good practice. Self-leadership defines that you should not always wait to be led towards best practice, but that you should research it for yourself and share appropriately with your team. At an early stage of leadership it does not always follow that your ideas will be put into routine practice, but this should not discourage you from becoming better informed and disseminating your informed suggestions appropriately within your team or service.

A starting point for developing these early personal and professional qualities of self-management and self-leadership is asking yourself questions such as 'Why did I enter mental health nursing?' and 'What do I expect to be doing when I am in a practice environment?' Basing your practice on values and ethics is crucial to practice development and underpins clinical leadership (see also Chapters 2 and 3). Developing an awareness of your own values base, which then becomes translated into values-based practice, can often be uncovered by asking yourself questions such as (Box 8.3): 'If I were receiving care from a mental health nurse, what would I expect from them?', 'What are my beliefs about people who become mentally unwell?' and 'How do I think people experiencing mental health difficulties should be treated?' Many of the issues around self-efficacy, values-based practice and service user perspectives are explored in Part 1 of this book.

Reflective Exercise 8.14

Ask yourself the questions raised in the last paragraph. Answer them as honestly as you are able, even though you may find that your answers are unsettling. Translating beneficent values into actions is an important part of nurse leadership.

Box 8.3

Service user experience: what do I want from my mental health nurse?
Note: this links to Chapters 1 and 17 in Barker (2009).

* 'A friendly ear, someone to talk to about my problems and who listens without judging me.'

* 'Someone to expound on my experience to, someone that gives me time to talk through my experience.'

- 'It's so useful to have someone who will give you time to talk out your problems with as when it is all in my head I get distressed and I can't concentrate, and then I need someone that I can "talk it out of my head" with.'

- 'To be available and easy to get hold of, or failing that someone who will get back to me when they say they will. And to know that when I call them it's because I need their support and times are difficult for me.'

- 'I want someone who is compassionate – but not too much! I want them to take the time to find out how I feel.'

- 'I want to be treated with dignity and respect – I don't feel I have always been, especially when I was at my most unwell, and remembering that is distressing. I don't want to be looked at and for someone to think "there's no point in talking to you as you aren't getting any better", keep trying because it does help me even when I am too unwell to respond properly – at least I feel noticed and that can be my turning point.'

- '… a proper amount of time to talk over problems.'

- 'I want my nurse to be well informed about mental health problems and treatments.'

- 'I like their informality, it helps you to relax with them.'

- 'It's not what you wear or how you look, you can tell when people are genuine – it's about the way they look at you and talk to you and make you feel at ease.'

- '… friendly attitude. If they are too demanding or attacking or even aggressive when you first meet them, because your head is all over the place, it makes you clam up and become more stressed, this approach is detrimental.'

Explicit verbal consent to present this information in an anonymized form for secondary purposes of education adhering to the NMC and British Association for Behavioural & Cognitive Psychotherapies (BABCP) professional codes. Thanks to M, J, S and C.

Reflective Exercise 8.15

Reflect on the information in Box 8.3.

- Were you surprised by the service users' comments?
- What themes can you pick out from their comments?
- What messages do they give you about how to undertake your role of mental health nurse?
- Reflect on self-leadership and self-management; what do these concepts mean to you?
- What factors and behaviours does it encompass?
- What would it mean to you personally and professionally to develop and adhere to these identified behaviours?
- What would it mean to mental health service users?

If we return to the developmental journey illustrated in Figure 8.3, we can see that at the same time as developing self-leadership and self-management you will be required to be developing the skills to manage and lead on individualized episodes of care. In pre-registration you will be academically taught and clinically mentored as part of this learning journey. As part of your practice experience you will become familiar with the governance requirements and policies that you are expected to adhere to for the management aspects of the care episode. To lead and manage individual care you need to be leading and managing yourself as a mental health nurse. You will need to have developed an understanding of your own values and of your attitude towards and beliefs about mental health difficulties and people who experience them; these factors combine to determine how you approach providing mental health care. In addition to this you will need to develop knowledge and understanding about mental health disorders and competency in talking therapeutically with service users to gain a more phenomenological picture of their experience. Depression is not just low mood, it is how living with low mood impacts on your life. You will also have to learn about guidelines and recommendations for best treatments.

Case Study 8.2 details an extensive learning opportunity (Reflective Exercise 8.16) to emphasize the understanding of leading and managing individualized care as part of your development journey.

Case Study 8.2

Leading and managing individualized care
Note: this links to Chapters 1, 15 and 17 in Barker (2009).

Marie is 34 years old. She has just been discharged from a brief inpatient stay and has been allocated you as her care co-ordinator. Marie has been experiencing low mood for about three years, she is married with two children, a son of five and a daughter of two years of age. Her admission was precipitated by Marie's increasing distress at believing she was unable to cope with the demands of her life. Marie currently tells you that she continues to feel low and scared, and complains of difficulties with her concentration. She tells you she is extremely tired even though she is in bed for up to 14 hours a day. After Marie drops her son off at school she retreats to her home, not leaving again until it is time to pick him up. She has no close friends and avoids other mothers in the playground as 'talking to people is just too much – I have nothing to say to them'.

Reflective Exercise 8.16

- What do you think the mental health nurse role needs to be for Marie?
- What do you think Marie's primary diagnosis is and what does this tell you about what Marie might be experiencing? How will her experience impact on your therapeutic relationship? How will you address these difficulties?

- What do best practice guidelines say about effective interventions for Marie?
- What elements would you expect to see in a collaborative nursing assessment of Marie's current experience?
- In order to lead this episode of care effectively, what do you need from yourself and from your team?

Role play: In groups of three, select one to be Marie, one to be the mental health nurse, and one an observer. Spend 20 minutes role playing a collaborative nursing assessment, developing a shared understanding, identifying two major problems, setting goals and detailing how you will work together to achieve them.

As the developmental journey continues around both hemispheres, it can be seen that the next steps to leadership and management competency attainment are to evaluate the individual episodes of care you have been leading and managing and utilize the information to consider care quality improvements. Such quality improvement can be small; for example, modifying an individual care package, or adjusting the therapeutic approach to a small group of service users with similar needs. Leading and managing smaller tasks successfully will develop your confidence to step forward to lead in wider spheres. An example of leading a care 'area' is offered in Case Study 8.3.

Case Study 8.3

Leading and managing a care area – developing the Living with Psychosis Support Group

In 2004 the psychosis service was becoming more aware of the issues around the experience of hearing distressing voices. The clinical intervention at that time for all service users with this experience was through individual cognitive behavioural therapy. There was a growing evidence base that therapeutic groups offered a benefit to people experiencing psychosis. This was complemented by the growth of the UK Hearing Voices Network, which was offering information from voice hearers that meeting with other voice hearers was supportive and psychologically beneficial. At the same time, the NHS Trust within which the psychosis service operates was pushing for the implementation of the NICE (2002) guideline for schizophrenia within which were recommended best treatment guidelines for persistent psychosis. The service called an open meeting of service users who were experiencing voices and discussed this growing evidence and knowledge with them. The service users were asked what they would like the psychosis service to do, and subsequently the Hearing Voices Group was set up by the psychosis service. This group continues to run today, now as the Living with Psychosis Support Group.

Reflective Exercise 8.17

- Think about a mental health practice environment that you are familiar with.
- Identify an improvement or addition to practice that you believe might benefit the team or the service users? How would you inform yourself about the evidence base that supports your idea? Develop an outline plan about how you would lead and manage this idea.
- Referring to Figure 8.1 think about how your development would impact on the different domains. Refer to Figure 8.2 and reflect on how you would lead the development within each domain and how you would engender support from each.

The developmental journey ends with roles in mental health service management and development. Not all nurses will wish to follow this journey to complete the circle, and nor should all nurses do so. The important point is to know that leadership and management are functions we undertake throughout the whole of our nursing career, and that the starting point of this journey is ourselves, on day 1 of our career in mental health nursing.

Summary

- Leadership and management are pivotal tasks for the nurse role.
- Leadership and management can be delineated in terms of tasks and roles but there are areas of overlap.
- Leaders and followers have a reciprocal relationship.
- Developing followership skills is as important as developing leadership skills.
- The journey of competency development in nurse leadership and management can be started from pre-registration and continued throughout your professional career.
- Self-leadership and self-management are essential skills in the developmental pathway.

Further reading

Barker P (1999) *The Philosophy and Practice of Psychiatric Nursing: Selected Writings.* London: Churchill Livingstone.
Barker P, Campbell P, Davidson B (eds) (2000) *From the Ashes of Experience: Reflections on Madness, Survival and Growth.* London: Whurr.

Romme M, Escher S, Dilllon J, Corstens D, Morris M (2009) *Living with Voices: 50 Stories of Recovery*. Ross-on-Wye: PCCS Books Ltd.

Sullivan EJ, Garland G (2010) *Practical Leadership and Management in Nursing*. Harlow: Pearson Education Ltd.

References

Adair J (2002) *Effective Strategic Leadership*. London: Palgrave MacMillan.

Alimo-Metcalfe B (2003) Leadership stamp of greatness. *Health Service Journal* **113**(5861), 28–32.

Barker P (ed.) (2009) *Psychiatric and Mental Health Nursing: The Craft of Caring*, 2nd edn. London: Hodder Arnold.

Bass BM (1985) *Leadership and Performance*. New York, NY: Free Press.

Brooker C, Brabban A (2004) *Measured Success: A Scoping Review of Evaluated Psychosocial Interventions Training for Work with People with Serious Mental Health Problems*. Mansfield: National Institute for Mental Health in England/Trent Workforce Development Confederation.

Burns JM (1978) *Leadership*. New York, NY: Harper and Row.

DH (2000) *The NHS Plan*. London: HMSO.

Harper J (1995) Clinical leadership – bridging theory and practice. *Nurse Education* **20**(3), 11–12.

Henderson A, Winch S (2008) Commentary. Managing the clinical setting for best nursing practice: a brief overview of contemporary initiatives. *Journal of Nursing Management* **16**, 92–5.

Hope R (2004) *Ten Essential Shared Capabilities*. London: Department of Health.

Marchionni C, Ritchie J (2008) Organizational factors that support the implementation of a nursing best practice guideline. *Journal of Nursing Management* **16**, 266–74.

Mullally S (2001) Leadership and politics. *Nursing Management* **8**(4), 21–7.

NICE (2002) *Schizophrenia: Core Interventions in the Treatment and Management of Schizophrenia in Primary and Secondary Care*. London: National Institute for Health and Clinical Excellence.

NMC (2010) *Standards of Competencies for Pre-registration Nurses*. London: Nursing and Midwifery Council.

Northouse PG (2004) *Leadership: Theory and Practice*, 3rd edn. London: Sage.

Pullen ML (2003) Developing clinical leadership skills in student nurses. *Nurse Education Today* **23**, 34–9.

RCN (2003) *Defining Nursing*. London: Royal College of Nursing.

Stanley D (2006) Recognizing and defining clinical nurse leaders. *British Journal of Nursing* **15**(2), 108–11.

Stanley D (2008) Congruent leadership: values in action. *Journal of Nursing Management* **16**, 519–24.

UKCC (1994) *The Future of Professional Practice: The Council's Standards for Education and Practice Following Registration: Position Statement on Policy and Implementation.* London: UKCC (now the Nursing and Midwifery Council).

Whitehead DK, Weiss SA, Tappen RM (2007) *Essentials of Nursing Leadership and Management*, 4th edn. Philadelphia, PA: EA Davis Co.

Wiggins MS, Hyrkäs K (2011) Achieving excellence in nursing management. *Journal of Nursing Management* **19**, 1–4.

CHAPTER NINE

Marion Aslan and Mike Smith

Promoting health and social inclusion

Learning outcomes

- Be able to demonstrate a critical understanding of the theory and practice of promoting health and inclusion
- Articulate an understanding of the politics, ethics and history of mental health care and exclusion
- Be able to critically evaluate the concept of thriving

Introduction

> *It is no measure of health to be well adjusted to a profoundly sick society.*
>
> *(Krishnamurthi 1975)*

Promoting health and inclusion are two concepts that are often rolled together. Why, one may ask? Because, when one considers the concepts of health and wellness, the issue of social inclusion and exclusion, as a citizen, becomes an essential consideration. This is even more pertinent when we consider and explore the concepts of 'recovery' and 'thriving'. In this chapter, we will argue that the history of psychiatry and of mental illness is primarily an issue of politics and citizenship. We acknowledge that not all mental health professionals share our politicized understanding of psychiatry as a history of exclusion, but perhaps we need to remember that the recovery movement originates not only in the field of mental illness, but also from groups of people excluded from society and demanding emancipation. The aim of this chapter is to therefore highlight the way in which the history of psychiatry can be read as a history of exclusion in order to fully understand what social inclusion means.

We will first consider promoting inclusion. For most of us, if we have not had the lived experience of being excluded at the state, societal and political level then considering the issues of inclusion is not something we do every day. Inclusion is a word that usually only gets used when others observe an individual or a group being overtly excluded – 'Include Johnny in the games' for example. Our observations and experiences of 'service user' inclusion illustrate this point. The person with lived experience is 'included' in policy meetings as a deliberate act, albeit as frequently to 'tick the box of inclusion' as to give meaningful opinions.

We cannot look at inclusion without first considering why we still today exclude people. In order to understand this, we need to consider the concepts of madness and mental illness and the historical origins and purpose of exclusion.

Reflective Exercise 9.1

Think of a time when you were excluded.

- At what level were you excluded?
- Was it temporary?
- Was it by peers or by people in positions of power?

Imagine that the people excluding you are the very offices of the country or state you live within, the government. Imagine this was done for 'your own good', but you disagreed with them, how would you feel and what might happen over time?

Exclusion from society: a view from history

The history of madness, its emergence, is well written about but we will highlight four simplified movements in social policy.

1. The creation of the madman as a beast.
2. The creation of the moral defective – Victorian era.
3. The creation of the different and the eugenics movement – post Victorian.
4. The creation of the mentally sick and diseased – post Second World War.

Bedlam or more correctly The Bethlem Hospital developed in the early sixteenth century as a consequence of the emerging social policy toward the insane. The

Bethlem Hospital in London is commonly held to be the first psychiatric hospital in the industrially developing world at that time. Equivalent structures were exported by the British powers and governments to our colonies and the 'colonization of madness' and the 'globalization of psychiatry' can be thought of as contributing to processes of cultural imperialism (Fernando 2010; Gilbert 1999). Madness in society was seen as the loss of reason, and it was reason that elevated us above the base level of the animal and differentiated between the animal and the human. The mad were therefore seen and regarded as no better than the beasts. They were treated the way some may treat beasts. They were locked and chained, and the places of the mad were seen as no different from circuses – arenas to view the beasts. The beatings and humiliation of the insane are well documented. It is important to consider that, once the concept of 'the beast' was established in our history, the treatment was to break them like the wild animals they were, so people were not just on view and paraded but the very treatment offered to them at the birth of psychiatry was to beat them and break them to help restore humanity. Although this makes for uncomfortable reading, we must recognize our history if we are to learn from it at all. We will ask you later to reflect on today's mental health care in the context of the history of mental health and ask you whether it is different or still fundamentally about inhumanity and exclusion. That is, are we as progressive as we think? This reflective opportunity is developed further in Chapter 10.

Bleedings, emetics, purgatives, beatings and pain became the agents of the animal master in Bethlem and as other mad people began to enter the asylum – the workless, the unwanted wife, the troublesome relative – the madhouses extended and were rebuilt. The role of the physician developed, and in 1774 it was the physician who certified whether a person was insane (The Madhouses Act 1774). Doctors soon became the arbiters of madness and sanity, with the instantaneous power and authority that this brought. They have remained in this position today despite many seminal works which question this authority and its credibility (see Rosenhan 1973). The fundamental principles of 'modern' mental health legal systems still rely upon the assessment of the loss of reason and the ability to function and reason autonomously (Mental Capacity Act 2005).

Reflective Exercise 9.2

Access Rosenhan's (1973) original papers or watch the videos on YouTube of David Rosenhan speaking about the original studies and his conclusions. With your fellow learners discuss what you feel were the key points and critical issues that arise from Rosenhan's study. Ask yourselves why psychiatrists attacked Rosenhan as unprofessional, rather than learning from what he had found.

Approaches to treating mental illness

With the madness of King George III and his subsequent recovery, many physicians began to tout their unique methods to cure the insane, and inducing hypothermia, near-drowning and other treatments began to replace the beatings (Whitaker 2002). Because these treatments were perceived to be beneficial, the physicians now working in 'madhouses' had to have a framework to explain why they were successful. The Royal Colleges were established and we see the beginning of movements for physicians to obtain social credibility as scientists rather than priests or mystics. This therefore was part of the overall social development of theories of cause and effect of mental illness as society began to root its beliefs in what became known as scientific 'method'. The development of the first organized resistance from victims of this treatment is often sourced to this Bedlam era. Nathaniel Lee (1649–92), for example, 'the mad poet' is often credited as a founder of resistance and we can see here a paraphrased version of his appeal in his petition for release.

They said I was mad and I said they were mad, damn them they outvoted me!

(Porter 2004)

The terms 'vapours', 'melancholy' and 'mania' entered clinical use and many brutal treatments became widespread. The assumption that mania was caused by the rush of blood to the head resulted in bleeding and bloodletting as treatments. Sadness was thought to be caused by too little blood to the head and was therefore treated by being spun in a chair to cause blood to rush to the brain. This too reflected wider medical practice where the humours (melancholic or black bile theories) were doctored and then the sanguine or blood theories became dominant in physical ailments (Porter 2004).

Pinel in France (during the French revolution), and Benjamin Rush and the Quakers (in the UK) began to question the brutality and high mortality rates in such 'treatment'. Pinel went as far as asserting that what was commonly viewed as madness was mostly the protestations of the inmates at the inhumanity of their treatment. From these writings and movements came a social change against the inhumanities that medical science had brought. This movement became known as 'moral treatment' in the UK and was the backbone of our policies until the early twentieth century. In 1796, after the death in 1791 of Hannah Mills (a Quaker and congregation member in the York Asylum), the Quakers and Tuke opened what was to become the York Retreat. The guiding principle of the retreat was that of Quakerism, that is, that we are all brethren and therefore we must treat people as brethren not beasts. Food, parties, social gatherings, kindness and quiet contemplation were all aspects of moral treatment. Even today, all who remember working in the then aged asylums recall the large ballrooms, the beautiful landscapes and gardens, the cricket pavilion, the farm and work, all key aspects of the approach (Hervey 1986; Nolan 1992).

> **Reflective Exercise 9.3**
>
> Think of our current work in psychiatry.
>
> - Can we still see any vestiges of moral treatment today?
> - Have you met older staff who have worked in the dying days of the old asylums?
> - How have they described the asylum with its ballrooms?
> - Do they have fond or regretful memories?
>
> Consider the proposition that when we closed the asylums perhaps we closed our hearts to suffering and opened our brains to science. If so, is it better today than it was in the nineteenth century?

Introduction of moral treatment

The Quakers did not bring about this change by revolution and protest but by just doing it differently themselves and by creating an alternative system to the monster that they thought psychiatry had become. Today a number of progressive and alternative organizations are also concluding that change will only come about by the creation of an alternative system rather than by trying to sanitize and change the one that we have. Interestingly, it is often the very fact of handpicked 'service user inclusion' by some mainstream organizations that is the catalyst for these alternative and progressive groups forming. The sentiment that 'We are all equal but some are more equal than others' becomes the impetus for change.

The Quakers wrote that all can recover but said that not all will, and for those who do not wish to or are unable to recover they offered a moral, humble and human support in a pleasant place of asylum. Of people who newly presented at the York Retreat, 70 per cent recovered, and of the chronically ill deemed incurable who were sent there, 25 per cent subsequently recovered (Whitaker 2002). By the 1840s, however, medicine had begun to reassert itself within the asylums and was administered alongside the moral treatment philosophies and environments. Alongside the distressed in the asylums were added further groups of people with dementia, syphilis, alcohol and drug problems, and we saw the decline of moral treatment. Money, financial restraints and the difficulty of recruiting kind staff on poor wages all added to a long deterioration of the moral asylum and the discrediting of moral treatment (Nolan 1998).

What Whitaker (2002) calls the darkest hour was now to follow. In terms of exclusion, 1900–50 was the most important and forgotten era. It was an era of genetics, eugenics and genocide that led to the organized and state-sanctioned murder of those deemed to be different in Hitler's Germany (Hitler 1930). In the UK, prior to the world war of 1939 we were not that far away from either America or Germany in the way science and medicine were leading us or in how we treated the mentally ill. This was an era of 'hard science' over the artisanship of the moral era and of medicine as the new religion and the cure for all ills. It is the era of modern mental health nursing and it is a part of our history that we need to acknowledge (Berghs *et al.* 2007; Nolan 1998).

This era ended with the revelations of genocide in Germany and the realization that many of the concentration camps had previously been psychiatric hospitals and the inmates had been among the first to be murdered in the name of science and eugenics. After Darwin's essays, Galton (1883) led the rise of the genetics lobby in British society. With genetics came the principle of selective advantage and of the ill, as they were becoming labelled, having a sickness that was permanent and to be eradicated from the evolutionary pool. Of course we know that the hole in this theory (apart from its ethical implications) is whether madness can be identified as a discrete entity. Can we define it? Do we know what it is and is it a negative trait?

Reflective Exercise 9.4

Many historical characters have been said to have taken inspiration rather than struggle from their supposed mental illness (Joan of Arc, Henry VI, Nietzsche). Search the internet to see if you can find examples of inspiration or behaviour in celebrities or famous people that could in some contexts be constructed as illness.

Exclusion

Because of the history described above, we have assumed that madness is a weakness that needs to be eradicated. The USA formally led the way with the Supreme Court being asked to rule in 1926 on whether a woman (note the politics of gender) could be compulsorily sterilized to prevent her passing the weakness of madness on to the next generation. The Court agreed with this proposition and thus eugenics was formalized by a state. Some would argue that Hitler's Germany and the National Socialists merely added organization and a widened definition as to what was seen to be weakness (Hitler 1930).

The British part of this history of exclusion was no better. Henry Maudsley was an eminent physician and founder of modern psychiatry in the UK (The Bethlem Hospital became named after him) who saw the origins of insanity in the family stock: the strain which, as the old saying goes, runs in the blood, but which we prefer now to describe as a fault or flaw in the germ-plasm passing by continuity of substance from generation to generation. Maudsley was a brilliant physician who withdrew from psychiatry in later life and often in his later presentations and private letters expressed regret at his career choice in psychiatry. Perhaps the greatest abuses of this time came with the development of psychosurgery, electroconvulsive therapy and malaria therapy, which often had fatal results and certainly long-term effects.

Reflective Exercise 9.5

Think about the practices and policies in Nazi Germany and what is now commonly known as the Holocaust. Think about the roles of nurses, doctors and hospitals in this process; for more specific papers, see Berghs *et al.* (2007).

With the revelations following the Nuremberg trials and the fall of the National Socialists, Europe and America had to rethink this history and we thus saw the birth of what we argue is 'modern exclusion'. The advent of the *Diagnostic and Statistical Manual of Mental Disorders* (DSM) and especially the changes from DSM-III to DSM-IV and the latest incarnation of DSM-IV are commonly seen as medical and scientific advances and great leaps forward in thinking; but they raise the following important questions:

1. Why are marginalized groups still disproportionately represented among the mentally ill groups (Littlewood and Lipsedge 1989)?
2. Have we moved on from the language of the 'beast' or do we just use current and modern language to infer the same meaning?
3. Is mental illness still primarily about separating 'us from them'?
4. Do we believe it can happen to anyone or are we different?
5. Why are recovery rates so low and disability rates so high in this era of scientific enlightenment (Warner 1994)?
6. Why is living in an industrially developed society a predictor of poor outcome from psychiatric diagnosis in a World Health Organization (WHO) study (Leff 1992)?
7. Is mental illness a biologically correct term or does it just sanitize and modernize exclusion?
8. Are today's scientific theories in psychiatry merely a reflection of wider medical treatments and theories being forced or shoehorned into psychiatry as an attempt to accrue social and scientific respectability?
9. Is most of what we do still based on basic theories of the medicalization of difference?
10. Are early deaths among psychiatric patients today a modern version of the old inhumanity and carelessness about the mentally ill?

Reflective Exercise 9.6

Read Ballasteros *et al.* (2000), Joukamaa (2006), and Harrow and Jobe (2007) for a discussion of the questions raised above.

Search the national media for half an hour or read a selection of popular magazines, and look for references to mental illness in society.

- How much of the reporting is positive?
- How much is about medicalizing a disease or finding a cure?
- How much of it is about excusing bad behaviour or labelling wrong or bad behaviour as mental illness?

Social inclusion

If people have been excluded and are to now be included, what are they to be included in? And how? Social inclusion is a rather generic term to describe including people back in to society who have been excluded from it for some reason and to varying degrees.

'Social inclusion' is often used as the antithesis of 'social exclusion'. 'Social cohesion' is a more recent term, but one which is increasingly being used across government as a theme joining up different aspects of its work.

(Charities Commission 2008)

The starting point for many, then, is to prevent exclusion and many new systems of health care provision are now targeting this area. Early intervention services in mental ill health aim generally to intervene early and in primarily non-medical ways to prevent a person who is newly distressed to not lose links that are crucial to recovery. Safe housing, work and good relationships are commonly known as the most reliable predictors of recovery, and services aim to retain these links as an easier option to having to restore them once lost. It is a costly model in the short term as it requires intensive short-term support across several domains of life such as working, education and a variety of issues in wellbeing such as building on strengths, finding positive futures and developing resilience and wellbeing.

Mental illness is still often constructed in social and political terms as being primarily about creating difference and excluding the different, as we saw in the beginnings of this chapter. The historical context of the development of asylums and the medicalization of difference and, more latterly, distress has to be fundamentally considered by all students working within this field. Mental health workers do not often consider this history and it is easy to oversimplify and medicalize a person's distress when you meet with them. We know that things may initially appear crazy and bizarre, but once we understand the context that they occur within (and time, engagement and relationship building often bring this context to us) they can actually start to appear meaningful and as metaphors for what is troubling someone. The craziness of the behaviour often disappears as we start to understand why the person is reacting in a specific way and we generally begin to see the whole person in context of the sum of their experiences.

Many people with lived experience of mental health problems, as part of their journey of recovery, begin to ask questions that it can take some workers many years to consider.

- Do people not have a right to be different and to think and feel differently (Shermer 1997)?
- Why is engagement in psychiatry always on the terms of those in power (not on the terms of the client)? For instance many consumers and their support circles feel that they have to agree with the mental illness worker's view to be seen as engaging with them or the system. Any differences in views is seen as being non-compliant or difficult.

- Why are clients' own explanations of their experiences often invalidated and reduced to concepts rooted in a singularly medical model or illness concept, such as 'You lack insight'? Why is this not seen as 'lazy practice' on behalf of the worker for failing to develop a construct?

The legal responsibilities and processes surrounding mental ill health are generally about the lawful conditions of exclusion and how we remove peoples' due rights and how we interfere with peoples' liberties on grounds of 'illness' (Mental Health Act 2007). They are not about inclusion and the restoration of wellness or the protections of citizens' rights for those people considered to be mentally ill. Some approaches to inclusion are necessarily person centred, but they see mental health difficulties residing between people (Beutler and Malik 2002). Social inclusion approaches see the wider social consequences of the experience of mental ill health and address issues of politics and work within this wider context. Jobs, meaningful occupation and social restoration become the wider areas of focus; and on an individual level, resourcefulness, wellness, resilience, interdependence and finding your lust for life and energy, and reclaiming self are areas of working focus.

It is difficult sometimes for workers to move forwards from the distress of the person in front of them to see the wider political aspects of exclusion and inclusion in modern society, but the following reflections may be helpful for you to clarify your views and values and to identify areas of your practice that you may wish to develop.

Reflective Exercise 9.7

- In today's more humane and medicalized times, why are life expectancies of psychiatric patients so much lower than the rest of the population?
- Why are recovery rates in the UK lower now than they were 100 years ago?
- Why are the outcomes so much better in Africa and Asia than in the industrialized and wealthier West?
- What, if anything, can we learn from African and Asian society about exclusion, inclusion, resilience and wellness (Leff 1992)?
- Why are society, mental health professionals and science dismissive of the criticisms about the validity of psychiatric concepts of mental illness (Boyle 1990)?

Promoting health and wellness

Health is more than just managing symptoms and restoration. The WHO (1948) definition of health is 'a state of complete physical, mental and social wellbeing and not merely the absence of disease or infirmity'. According to the WHO (1986) we promote wellness not just by dealing with disease but by addressing the structural issues (such as discrimination, poverty and unemployment) that affect our health and the choices we make, as well as focusing on the knowledge and behaviour of individuals or groups of people.

Many approaches to recovery have fallen into similar traps, where they are readily co-opted, especially by states and services, to mean merely the management of symptoms and preventing relapse. Symptom management and relapse prevention, for some, are of course part of getting stable, which in itself is an early part of the recovery journey, but it is not usually an end in itself and indeed it can be a place where many get 'stuck' and never move on from (Aslan and Smith 2009). This is frequently a consequence of groups of people either not fully understanding the elements and core values of recovery, not being willing to change ideas or practice or rejecting the philosophy of true recovery.

Recovery used to mean what we now call thriving and it is consistent with working, contributing to your society, enjoying life and being undetectably ever a patient (Whitaker 2010). Recovery should mean far more than the outdated diluted view that it is a 'growing mastering of illness management with resultant reduction of symptoms' (Aslan and Smith 2007, p.6). There are great dangers with altering the concepts in order to widen their appeal – hence the use of more dynamic terms such as thriving because they are difficult to dilute (see Aslan and Smith 2007).

Preventing breakdown

We need, as workers, to have an understanding of the process of breakdown and its consequences for the client and their social networks in order to understand how we may support and help the individual to prevent or limit the descent into breakdown.

Erving Goffman, the Canadian sociologist, in his seminal (1961) work wrote of the process of 'stripping' as the way that the process of breakdown affects the individual. He describes how the process of breakdown, and the way society responds to it, strips the person of simple things such as responsibility, then identity, then citizenship and self. There is no doubt that for some people the removal of responsibility and the role of nurse or mental health worker as expert can be helpful and beneficial. But any removal of liberty, responsibility and self-direction must be temporary and for as short a period as possible. The restoration of self is often written about in survivor literature as essential in beginning the struggle to retain identity and self-determination. Words used historically to recognize this are convalescence, nurturing, helping, handing over, allowing temporary shutdown.

A key feature in preventing breakdown involves recognizing when someone is overwhelmed. That is, we can all be resilient and strong, and we try to strive to survive but often the weight of our burdens are too great. Hence for a worker to remove this burden temporarily may be therapeutic and desperately needed. Sometimes the factors that conspire against us in our efforts to deal with these burdens are too great and 'toxic', and therefore the most useful role for workers at this stage is to help in removing toxic factors and to offer ideas to increase someone's natural coping strategies in order to help to build resilience. As stated previously, the concepts of early intervention tend to be very assertive and resourceful within these areas and aim to prevent the descent into disintegrative ego states and states of dependence and disability.

We mentioned briefly before about what might seem like craziness and finding a context for it. When people's lives are collapsing they may try to find ways of resuming control and function, or try to block out difficulties in whatever way they can. A common strategy many of us may use, for example, is alcohol. When alcohol takes the edge off, helps us forget or cope, it serves a purpose. If it starts to then cause more difficulties than it is helping with, drinking alcohol is seen as problematic and a symptom of illness. In the same way, people may 'choose' or find themselves using a different strategy – self-harm, voice hearing, depression, mania, psychosis. Initially this is the messenger that something is wrong, but over time it soon comes to be seen as the symptom of a particular disorder, rather than as a message to be understood. Instead of seeing a person trying to cope with distress we see the mad person, the 'beast', the 'other'. Workers can assist by helping the person understand the messenger within the context of their life experiences, particularly where this has involved trauma. In this way we start to promote understanding and breakthrough.

For some people (for example, the individual in Case Study 9.1) their 'distress' may in fact have a spiritual, religious or esoteric message embedded in it.

Case Study 9.1

'Perhaps the most poignant episode of voices was just before Easter time in 2002 when once again I ended up on a legal detainment. For no reason that I could think of a spiritual voice in my head was telling me I needed to be in the village where my father grew up, get involved with the village community in some way, that it was an important place for me. I started spending time at the local pub and got to know quite a few people, and before I knew what I was letting myself in for had agreed to buy a horse, put my house on the market and was planning to move out to the village. At the same time I was more and more listening to my spiritual guide, working hard, eating and sleeping little, and eventually I burned out. My family were concerned, called in the crisis team and much against my will I was once again in hospital. The staff viewed my voice hearing as a symptom of psychosis so I tended not to share much with them and kept myself to myself.

'During my stay, brief as always, thankfully, I listened to a new voice that came in immediately I was admitted, that of my father (still alive and, although in his early eighties, healthy and active). In reality he would visit me during the day,

continued ➤

but when he and my mother left his "voice" would return to be with me constantly. We had long conversations and "discussed" much about life and dying, it felt that he was preparing me for his death and the conversations were as real to me as any I'd ever had with him. They lasted for several days then disappeared, and I returned home within the week.

'Although I eventually decided not to move, and had to return the horse to its owner six months later, I spent many happy days recovering through riding through the countryside where my father had lived. He and my mother would sometimes accompany me and my son, going over old times, talking about his childhood and how the landscape had changed.

'My father's funeral was a year later on Good Friday. He had died very suddenly, no warning at all – a year to the day I had been sectioned.' (Aslan 2009)

Promoting breakthrough

When a person has reached depths of distress and human suffering, our role as workers is to support them to break through the problems and adversity that they find themselves within, enabling new growth and new futures (Laing 1967). The enemy at this stage is stability and maintenance, as, often, once a person gets themselves to a position of stability, it is hard to raise their own and other people's expectations for further work and aspiration. People internalize the 'this is as good as it gets' sentiments of others and systems can conspire to keep people stable at all costs especially when the person wants to stop engaging with services or move back on with their life. When a person has been to the depths of suffering and distress people are aware of their darkest times and are scared to push them too hard to breakthrough in case they take a step backwards. For workers therefore it might be important to establish confidence, support and plan in order to avoid these pitfalls. Backward steps or setbacks may also be inevitable and necessary. The restoration or more correctly reclamation of responsibility is critical for workers to support and enable at this stage; indeed, in some systems such as the 'open dialogue approach' this 'grip on life' is a major factor in clinical decision-making and risk-taking/management (Seikkula *et al.* 2003).

For the client, it becomes necessary to begin the rebuilding process as they progress within the breakthrough stage. Things that have been taken or removed from them, like responsibility and autonomy, become issues for them to address and to be supported with. Social relationships, building esteem, finding the functional self, finding new ways of coping and surviving that cause less harm all become the strategies and activities of the person in breakthrough. Understanding what it was that led us to the position of being overwhelmed and to breakdown is a difficult task but one that can be found in many stories of human growth from adversity (see Aslan 2008b).

> **Reflective Exercise 9.8**
>
> Seeking stability and/or feeling stuck is a human experience that is common and potentially entrapping to all of us. Think about a time in your relationships or working life when you have become 'stuck' and/or have accepted your lot as 'good enough'. Can you understand how this, for clients, is both a comfort for a time and possibly a necessary resting point, and also a potential threat and danger that can entrap and enslave them for the rest of their lives?

Aiming to break out

To break out is a personal and political act that is as self-inclusive as the construct of mental illness is socially exclusive. To become 'weller than well' as a result of prior distress and difficulty is often declared in the recovery and thriving literature. Karl Menninger *et al.* (1963) introduced the idea of recovery being a potentially transformational and liberating process. Menninger had an illustrious career in the science and medicalization of madness in the early part of the twenty-first century before apparently changing his mind about the medical approach:

> *Not infrequently we observe that a patient who is in a phase of recovery from what may have been a rather long illness shows continued improvement, past the point of his former 'normal' state of existence. He not only gets well, to use the vernacular; he gets as well as he was, and then continues to improve still further. He increases his productivity; he expands his life and its horizons. He develops new talents, new powers, and new effectiveness. He becomes, one might say, 'Weller than well.' ... every experienced psychiatrist has seen it ... What could it mean? It violates our conventional medical expectations, so perhaps it is often overlooked and occurs more often than we know ... ['it is obvious that] transcendence does occur.*
>
> (Menninger et al. 1963)

The concept of transcendence or transformational crisis is today frequently heard, spoken of by those who have moved beyond recovery and are thriving and who assert that their experiences were life-changing and not to be regretted. In fact, many would assert that they are glad they went through the experience to get to the place where they are today. In addition many assert that they were never ill in the first place!

Consumers or survivors of course cottoned on to this common-sense approach many years ago and Nathaniel Lee was not the only one presumed incurable in the asylums of the UK who spoke out, fought back and proved people wrong. Indeed Gale and Howard's (2003) book comprises collected assertions of the patients from the old Bethlem asylum archives of nineteenth- and twentieth-century Britain. Again, Irving Gottesman (1991) gives more contemporary accounts of people diagnosed with schizophrenia who defied the wisdom that this was an 'incurable disease' and who rejected the imposed view in order to break out and to demand inclusion.

Mental health and community workers cannot empower per se but they can create the conditions and the expectations that, regardless of exclusion, people can emancipate themselves. This requires the worker to understand the history and relevance of exclusion to the client and the battles that they have had and will have to first survive and then to move through to thrive.

Any practice dealing with inclusion has to understand how and on what levels people are excluded in order to be in a position to help. It is apparent that research and evidence in psychiatric practice is biased and politicized in many ways and at many levels (Boyle 1990; Caplan and Cosgrove 2004; Whitaker 2002). The concepts of who goes on to thrive, to be 'weller than well', has been subsumed by the body of evidence directed by drug and therapy industries to create distress as an illness or personal deficiency that can keep people in systems by portraying it as a chronic, hopeless condition, where the best you can hope for is to be stable and maintained. The emancipation section of the thrive manual (Aslan and Smith 2007) aims to assist workers and clients to become aware of the politics of exclusion and inclusion and to activate themselves to learn and grow with the help of others and via networks sharing information. Whitaker (2010) rightly points out how recovery used to be far more than what we see it as now. It used to involve working, leaving dependence and shunning concepts of disability. He sums up the issues best for American society by asserting simply that the wealthiest nation in the world cannot afford financially or morally the disability rates and levels of exclusion current mental illness policies have led us to.

Clinical and practice implications

As reflective practitioners working in modern times we need our history to inform our practice. When faced with individual recipients of our care and/or treatment it is easy to be seduced by short-term views, to believe that we are helping, whereas the long-term outcome statistics may indeed demonstrate some of our beliefs to be almost delusional!

The incidence of mental illnesses is increasing significantly. Bipolar disorder rates have changed from 1:5000 to 1:48 in the USA (Whitaker 2010) and recovery rates are dropping substantially. Some psychotic and mood disorders are now described as having changed to chronic rather than episodic. Disability rates are growing massively with morbidity and mortality rates increasing (Whitaker 2010). In these humane times, exclusion too is increasing. How many people who experience psychosis are in full gainful employment? How many own homes and how many hold active and valued roles in their communities?

We have no doubt progressed since the eighteenth century in terms of a move away from brutality and toward humanity, but we need to individually learn from that progression. Since the Second World War our focus on illness, treatment and pills has forced many mental health workers into situations where they feel that they lack holism, a key facet they would assert is necessary to their profession. Health and wellness practice must necessarily be holistic and person-centred and act against reductionist models of support that do not fit in with, or resonate with, client's wishes. Of course a paradox exists within mental health care and the craft of caring. This is the paradox of the legal framework we work within because of beliefs that clients may lack insight and are not able to make autonomous (in legal terms) judgements in the interests of their own health and wellbeing. First this issue needs to be seen in context; it only describes a minority of clients and must be seen as temporary and transient, within the legal frameworks of capacity. This issue is one of human rights, civil liberty and humanity and indeed in our eyes it is an issue about full citizenship that is promoted from within critical thinking networks.

It is worth referring back to one of the founders of the caring professions when she wrote the following about nursing:

The role of the nurse is to place the patient in the best position for nature to act upon him.

(Nightingale 1859)

The politics, ethics and history of mental health care are not substantial parts of basic education in clinical practice yet most reflective workers soon realize, as they struggle to develop their clinical competencies, that they are of utmost importance. Consumers and family members are often better educated in this history and these philosophical considerations than most workers. Their personal experience of a system, if it is not immediately helpful, is to find broader and more helpful solutions and strategies and of course the meaning and importance of doing this is far more significant to them than it might be to workers.

Repeated governments have tried to repeal and redraw completely the health law and there is a developing focus in mental health policy on illness prevention, health promotion and people progressing from situations of disability into employment and citizenship. Governments are becoming aware that our current policies which focus upon illness and disability have become or soon will be unaffordable given the growth in numbers of people with mental ill health. Government policy since 1999 has clearly been attempting to shift expenditure from illness models to health promotion and wellness models albeit slowly.

Reflective Exercise 9.9

Look at the following policy documents and see if there is an increasing emphasis on social inclusion:

* *The National Service Framework for Mental Health: Modern Standards and Service Models* (Department of Health (DH) 1999)
* *New Horizons: A Shared Vision for Mental Health* (DH 2009)
* *No Health Without Mental Health: A Cross Government Mental Health Outcomes Strategy for People of all Ages* (DH 2011).

Clearly, as you read these policies you will see that mental wellbeing is an issue for all of us. The UK government (as with other governments) is working towards concepts of wellbeing leading our policies rather than ones of illness and disability. The normalization of the experience of mental health problems in the wider community is positive and the focus on wellness and the restoration of wellbeing is a welcome policy direction. In latest policy, the government is beginning to focus not on treatments and therapies and activity but on outcomes. As we have seen above, current illness services in the National Health Service (NHS) and elsewhere in the UK do not have good outcomes and indeed on most outcome measures it is at best appalling. Ask yourself how many people in your service today are expected to quickly reclaim their lives and leave the service. How many people today are becoming 'disabled' as a result of mental ill health and being excluded from work and participation in community?

Stigma, both overt and internalized, is being positively addressed and many resources are freely available from government sources such as the anti-stigma toolkit (see http://www.chimat.org.uk/resource/view.aspx?QN=tacklingstigma). The (IAACM) was founded after Martin Luther King Junior said repeatedly that the world was in dire need of a new organization (see the International Association for the Advancement of Creative Maladjustment, http://www.mindfreedom.org/campaign/madpride/other-info/mlk-iaacm/iaacm-launched/?searchterm=iaacm). Many progressive and critical groups are learning from and deliberately politicizing madness and the politics of oppression in order to raise public awareness and to learn from movements in civil rights such as suffrage, racial equality and political imprisonment.

Focus on wellbeing and restoration

Most contemporary approaches to promoting recovery from distress and the restoration, and promotion, of wellbeing agree that an impulse towards human growth exists within us. This process is one of learning from adversity and developing skills to help one deal with future adversity in different ways in order that you do not go down the same path again. According to Einstein:

> *Insanity is: doing the same thing over and over again and expecting different results.*
>
> *(Rita Mae Brown 1983)*

In health restoration and inclusion services, the focus is upon relearning skills, reclaiming loss, building resilience and moving to wellness. It is about participating in communities, challenging stigma, raising public awareness and healing injury. Finally, it focuses on keeping safe, rebuilding personal responsibility, getting active and being dynamic.

Nursing and helping is about supporting, enabling and perhaps not getting in the way of the above activities where possible. Critical in this process is putting the client at the centre of this process, as it is their experiences, their lives and their wellness that we are supporting them with. People do need help and assistance at times in their lives. Specialist help from a professional with knowledge of the multitude of paths one can tread and the skills needed to go down each route can be a helpful resource for a client.

An example of the use of some of these inclusion philosophies in a modern mental health service is in the early intervention and active treatment of people in Northern Finland who experience psychosis and are at risk of becoming labelled over time with schizophrenia. The philosophy used is known as 'open dialogue' and it is an intensive treatment programme where psychiatric drugs are not used if possible (for as long as possible), and, if used, are discontinued when they are no longer needed and are regularly reviewed. This programme has had some outstanding results (see Seikkula *et al.* 2003).

Progressive philosophical approaches which have been used with positive results are the trialogue seminars and groups (mostly German-speaking countries) which have now been pioneered in the USA by Bock and Priebe (2005) and Amering *et al.* (2002).

Language and values

Our final reflections in this chapter are on the languages we use when we encounter the field of mental ill health. We still use language of difficulty and a primarily illness-focused language of deficit, dysfunction and hopelessness. This can only perpetuate a learned helplessness view of recovery, which in turn promotes an illness model and not a recovery approach. There are real dangers in using medicalized terminology to describe people's individual experiences, although understandably there are occasions when we utilize words in order to try to share a common understanding. Perhaps a more suitable terminology would be a 'different view of the world'. This rephrasing leads us automatically to reflect on 'whose view' we as nurses should be working with.

However there are some very simple alterations that we can all aspire to reflect on, change and put into practice, e.g. calling auditory hallucinations by the far more appropriate term of voice hearing. The former implies a medical condition, even a fictitious problem, while the latter describes the actual experience.

Reflective Exercise 9.10

List words that you have heard and/or used to describe your clients.

- Can you think of non-medical terminologies which better describe their experiences?
- If our language of distress serves to exclude people, how can it also allow for inclusion?

Conclusion

Perhaps in the same way that the term recovery has become all too frequently co-opted and assimilated into a maintenance model, we need to examine whether the term inclusion has similarly been corrupted. We can include people in a variety of settings yet not value their viewpoints; they may be regarded for their presence but not their prescience. Examples of this can be found in the User Movement, where individuals have been invited to policy groups, interview panels, boards of organizations etc. and when agreeing with the professionals are accepted as being experts of their experience yet immediately they challenge or 'rock the boat' they are ignored or overruled and seen to be lacking knowledge (Aslan 2008a). The following poem beautifully illustrates the point about inclusion becoming an organizational tokenistic duty and a valueless exercise rooted in target achievement.

Accolade

By Tessa Lowe

I arrived

At half-past-nine

Just in time

To receive my glossy certificate

Of appreciation

For having made a valuable contribution

To the august worry-tower event

How perceptively clairvoyant

They must have been

To have seen

So far in advance

That I would make

Such a valuable contribution

To the Alice-in-Wonderland proceedings

I could have been flattered

Had it not mattered

That every service user

Sorry

Every person with – mental-health-experiences

Received one too

What is a mentally healthy person

To do with such banal insanity

Such institutional insanity

Such seduction of one's vanity

Here's a valuable contribution

To your stinking unthinking
We're mad
Not stupid!

Unless mental health institutions and organizations that actively seek to 'include' those with a lived experience of distress move away from the tokenistic notions of inclusion, how can we expect society at large to move away from its notions of 'the beast' or 'the other'? In the same way that thriving throws down the gauntlet to us to reflect on our recovery practice, perhaps we need to start looking at 'integration' as being the benchmark of good practice in health promotion. By definition, integration is a more encompassing term:

- You are 'included' in the social network when you become part of it, accepting its rules and values
- You are 'integrated' if you can also act to modify rules and values of the social network – if you are an active actor and not only a passive member.

Further reading and useful websites

Goldacre B (2010) *The Stigma Gene.* Online: www.badscience.net/2010/10/pride-and-prejudice/#more-1801 (accessed 1 June 2011).
The Weller Than Well Research Project. Online: www.successfulschizophrenia.org/wtw.html (accessed 1 June 2011).
Online: www.crazydiamond.org.uk (accessed 1 June 2011).
Online: www.elemental.org.uk (accessed 1 June 2011).
Online: www.mindfreedom.org (accessed 1 June 2011).

References

Amering M, Hofer H, Rath I (2002) The 'First Vienna Trialogue' – experiences with a new form of communication between users, relatives and mental health professionals, in Lefley HP, Johnson DL (eds) *Family Interventions in Mental Illness: International Perspectives.* Westport, CT: Praeger.
Aslan M (2008a) *The Art of Thriving: Beyond Recovery.* Newton Le Willows: Crazy Diamond Publishing.
Aslan M (2008b) *From Recovery to Emancipation – Stories of Hope.* Newton Le Willows: Crazy Diamond Publishing.
Aslan M (2009) Introduction to the fifty stories, in Romme M, Escher S, Dillon J, Corstens D, Morris M (eds) *Living with Voices: An Anthology of 50 Voice Hearers Stories of Recovery.* Ross-on-Wye: PCCS Books.
Aslan M, Smith M (2007) *The Thrive Approach to Mental Wellness.* Newton Le Willows: Crazy Diamond Publishing.

Aslan M, Smith M (2009) *Overcoming Sadness and Depression*. Newton Le Willows: Crazy Diamond Publishing.

Ballesteros J, Gonzalez-Pinto A, Bulbena A (2000) Tardive dyskinesia associated with higher mortality rates in psychiatric patients: results of a meta-analysis of seven independent studies. *Journal of clinical Psychopharmacology* **20**, 188–94.

Berghs M, Dierckx De Casterle B, Gastmans C (2007) Practices of responsibility and nurses during the euthanasia programs of Nazi Germany, a discussion paper. *International Journal of Nursing Studies* **44**(5), 845–54.

Beutler L, Malik M (2002) *Rethinking the DSM: a Psychological Perspective*. Washington, DC: American Psychological Association.

Bock T, Priebe S (2005) Psychosis seminars: an unconventional approach. *Psychiatric Services* **56**(11), 1441–3.

Boyle M (1990) *Schizophrenia: a Scientific Delusion?* London: Routledge.

Brown RM (1983) *Sudden Death*. Westminster, MD: Bantam Books.

Caplan P, Cosgrove L (2004) *Bias in Psychiatric Diagnosis*. Lanham, MD: Jason Aronson.

Charities Commission (2008) *Draft Guidance for Consultation 'Social Inclusion'*. Online: www.charitycommission.gov.uk/Library/guidance/pbpsinc.pdf (accessed 1 June 2011).

DH (1999) *The National Service Framework for Mental Health: Modern Standards and Service Models*. London: Department of Health. Online: www.dh.gov.uk (accessed 1 June 2011).

DH (2009) *New Horizons: A Shared Vision for Mental Health*. London: Department of Health. Online: www.dh.gov.uk (accessed 1 June 2011).

DH (2011) *No Health Without Mental Health: A Cross Government Mental Health Outcomes Strategy for People of all Ages*. London: Department of Health. Online: www.dh.gov.uk (accessed 1 June 2011).

Fernando S (2010) *Mental Health Race and Culture*. London: Palgrave Macmillan.

Gale C, Howard R (2003) *Presumed Curable*. Petersfield: Wrightson Biomedical Publishing.

Galton F (1883) *Enquiries into Human Faculty and its Development*. London: JM Dent and Co.

Gilbert J (1999) Responding to mental distress: cultural imperialism or the struggle for synthesis? *Development in Practice* **9**(3), 287–95.

Goffman E (1961) *Asylums: Essays on the Social Situation of Mental Patients and Other Inmates*. New York, NY: Doubleday.

Gottesman I (1991) *Schizophrenia Genesis: The Origins of Madness*. New York, NY: WH Freeman and Co.

Harrow M, Jobe TH (2007) Factors involved in outcome and recovery in schizophrenia patients not on anti psychotic medications: A fifteen year multi follow-up study. *Journal of Nervous and Mental Diseases* **195**, 407–14.

Hervey N (1986) Advocacy or folly: the Alleged Lunatics' Friend Society, 1845–63. *Medical History* **30**(3), 245–75.

Hitler A (1930) *Mein Kampf Franz Eher Nachfolger*. Munich Franz Eher Machfolger.

Joukamaa J (2006) Schizophrenia, neuroleptic medication and mortality. *British Journal of Psychiatry* **188**, 122–7.

Krishnamurthi J (1975) *Freedom from the Unknown*. San Francisco, Harper.

Laing RD (1967) *The Politics of Experience and the Bird of Paradise*. London: Penguin.

Leff J (1992) The international pilot study of schizophrenia. *Psychological Medicine* **22**, 131–5.

Littlewood R, Lipsedge M (1989) *Aliens and Alienists, Ethnic Minorities and Psychiatry*. London: Unwin Hyman.

Menninger K, Mayman M, Pruyser P (1963) *The Vital Balance*. New York, NY: Vikin.

Mental Capacity Act (2005) Online: legislation.gov.uk/ukpga/2005/9/contents (accessed 1 June 2011).

Mental Health Act (2007) Online: legislation.gov.uk/ukpga/2007/12/contents/enacted (accessed 1 June 2011).

Nightingale F (1859) *Notes on Nursing: What Nursing is, What Nursing is Not*. London: Harrison & Sons.

Nolan P (1992) A history of the training of asylum nurses. *Journal* of *Advanced Nursing* **18**(8), 1193–201.

Nolan P (1998) *A History of Mental Health Nursing*. Cheltenham: Nelson Thornes.

Porter R (2004) *Madness: A Brief History*. Oxford: Oxford University Press.

Rosenhan DL (1973) *On Being Sane in Insane Places*. New York, NY: Science.

Seikkula J, Aaltonen J, Rasinkangas A, Alakare B, Holma J, Lehtinen V (2003) Open dialogue approach: treatment principles and preliminary results of a two-year follow-up on first episode schizophrenia. *Ethical and Human Sciences and Services* **5**(3), 163–82.

Shermer M (1997) *Why People Believe Weird Things*. New York, NY: WH Freeman and Co.

The Madhouses Act (1774) (14 Geo. 3 c.49).

Warner R (1994) *Recovery from Schizophrenia; Psychiatry and the Political Economy*. London: Routledge.

Whitaker R (2002) *Mad in America 'Bad Science, Bad Medicine and the Enduring Mistreatment of the Mentally Ill'*. Cambridge, MA: Perseus Publishing.

Whitaker R (2010) *Anatomy of an Epidemic, Magic Bullets, Psychiatric Drugs, and the Astonishing Rise of Mental Illness in America*. New York, NY: Random House.

WHO (1948) *Preamble to the Constitution of the World Health Organization as adopted by the International Health Conference*, New York, 19–22 June 1946; signed on 22 July 1946 by the representatives of 61 States (Official Records of the World Health Organization, no. 2, p. 100) and entered into force on 7 April 1948.

WHO (1986) *Health Promotion: Concepts and Principles in Action – A Policy Framework*. Copenhagen: World Health Organization Regional Office for Europe.

CHAPTER TEN

Diane Carpenter

The what then, what now and what next of mental health nursing

Learning outcomes

- Be able to critically analyse the 'histories' of mental health nursing and mental health care and treatment and evaluate these in their historical and contemporary contexts

- Think critically about the extent to which current mental health practice has been influenced by interpretations of the past

- Contribute meaningfully and critically to discussion about the future of the profession

Introduction

The Nursing and Midwifery Council code (NMC 2008) maintains that the public can be confident that new nurses will act on their understanding of how people's lifestyles, environments and the location of care delivery influence their health and wellbeing. The exercises in this chapter will encourage the critical thinking necessary to underpin this achievement. They will also help you achieve the following competencies detailed in the NMC (2010) standards for pre-registration in nursing:

- Mental health nurses must practise in a way that addresses the potential power imbalances between professionals and people experiencing mental health problems, including situations when compulsory measures are used, by helping people exercise their rights, upholding safeguards and ensuring minimal restrictions on their lives. They must have an in-depth understanding of mental health legislation and how it relates to care and treatment of people with mental health problems (p. 22).

- Mental health nurses must promote mental health and wellbeing, while challenging the inequalities and discrimination that may arise from or contribute to mental health problems (p. 23).

- Mental health nurses must work with people in a way that values, respects and explores the meaning of their individual lived experiences of mental health problems, to provide person-centred and recovery-focused practice (p. 23).

Barker (2009) focuses on the development of mental health nursing. How, he asks, 'might this "new world" of mental health nursing distinguish itself from the "old order" of psychiatric nursing?' And, 'how might nurses know when psychiatric or mental health nursing was indicated?' (pp. 3–8). Similarly he asks whether the emergent concept of 'recovery' is the final destination of care or the latest fashion soon to be replaced by another fad. In a reworking of Driscoll's model of reflective practice (1994), perhaps these questions can be addressed. Rather than considering the 'what, so what, and now what' of our individual clinical practice we might think about the 'what then, what now, what next' of our profession. Indeed we may also wish to review whether we have based the 'what now' on a misunderstanding or misinterpretation of the past, and, if so, whether any readjustments to our awareness of the history of our profession might alter the way we plan to care for the mentally ill in the future.

Gardner and Rolfe (2009) are historically sympathetic in their section on the 'war of the roses' (p. 670) and in their discussion of the possibility of genuine mental health nursing. They analyse the technological versus the humanist approaches of Kevin Gournay and Phil Barker (the former is an advocate for psychiatric nursing, the latter for mental health nursing) although they do not suggest who should be associated with which rose! To do so would have been to suggest a bias. But how important is the terminology we use? Do words define what we do? Does it matter what we do and what we are called? As Humpty Dumpty said in Lewis Carroll's *Through the Looking Glass* (1907):

'When I use a word,' Humpty Dumpty said, in rather a scornful tone, 'it means just what I choose it to mean — neither more nor less.'

'The question is,' said Alice, 'whether you **can** *make words mean so many different things.'*

'The question is,' said Humpty Dumpty, 'which is to be master — that's all.'

This chapter, therefore, raises questions about our understanding of the history of our profession and presents some challenges to the way in which we think about what we do now as a result of our historical sympathies. It addresses Barker's questions of therapeutic fads and also considers the consequences of nomenclature to current clinical practice. The examination of these dual aspects raises further questions about the future of nursing people with mental health problems. The chapter concludes by applying critical thinking about past and present practice to our personal future development as nurses, practitioners, therapists or whatever we choose to call ourselves.

The 'what then?' of mental health nursing

There is much debate about the use of history and historical sensitivity to contemporary life in whatever field it may arise. In 2003 the then British Prime Minister Tony Blair remarked in a speech to the United States Congress that 'there has never been a time ... when, except in the most general sense, a study of history provides so little instruction for our present day'. Yet when British troops entered Basra in April of that year, few people in Britain realized this had occurred before in 1914 (Tosh 2008). The circumstances were vastly different, but as George Santayana stated in 1905 'Those who cannot remember the past are condemned to repeat it' (Santayana 1920, p. 284). Tosh (2008) explains how lessons could have been learnt by reflecting on the 1914 invasion of Iraq and which might have altered the course of the conflict in 2003. There is a further problem with history, however. Despite attempts and claims to have achieved impartiality, no account of history is without its bias. Much of what we understand about the history of mental health nursing has been subject to the interpretation of the historian and many histories of our profession have been written by those with an interest in mental health, but without knowledge of the discipline of historical research. The debate rages here as well. Who is best placed to write the history of our profession: a practitioner with an interest in history or an historian with an interest in mental health? There are advantages and disadvantages in either case. Two prominent figures, however, have played a considerable part in shaping our history – Michel Foucault (a post-modern philosopher) and Andrew Scull (a Marxist sociologist) – neither of whom were historians or mental health practitioners of any description. In 1993 Peter Nolan, a prominent mental health nurse educator, published a history of mental health nursing. He wrote with a clear understanding of the recent history of the profession and contemporary mental health nursing within the scope his own experience of many years. However, he drew quite heavily on the work of Andrew Scull and others like him.

Foucault (2001, 2006) and Scull (1979) have focused on the incarceration and 'warehousing' of the mentally ill in their analyses of asylum care. Their views have considerable resonance with Erving Goffman's (a social anthropologist with an interest in mental health), who in 1961 wrote a book entitled *Asylums: Essays on the Social Situation of Mental Patients and Other Inmates*. Goffman berated the total institution that asylums provided. Indeed, in the same year that he published this seminal work, the Right Honourable J Enoch Powell, the Minister of Health, delivered his now famous 'Water Towers' speech culminating in:

> *There they stand, isolated, majestic, imperious, brooded over by the gigantic water tower and chimney combined, rising unmistakable and daunting out of the countryside – the asylums which our forefathers built with such immense solidity to express the notions of their day. Do not for a moment underestimate their powers of resistance to our assault.*
>
> (Speech at the annual conference of the National
> Association of Mental Health (now Mind), 1961)

There is a contemporary cult of people who break into disused asylums and take photographs of their dereliction to be published on websites, often with titles such as 'Sick Britain' (2009). In themselves such sites claim to present a photographic art form, but the implication, in keeping with the writings of Foucault and Scull, is that asylum care was unpleasant, unhelpful and inhumane. The problem with these interpretations is that they are anachronistic – they are taken out of appropriate historical context and bear the marks of those who do not understand the discipline of history. They with Goffman share a further criticism – that they generalized their analyses of their findings based on too little evidence, too few examples.

Further research (Carpenter 2010) has raised doubts about the generalizability of the inhumanity of incarceration with alternative examples. Carpenter argued that for the period of her study (1845–1914) asylum care, which provided principally for paupers, in many cases (although in all likelihood not exclusively) offered an improved quality of life than might have been found in the lunatic wards of workhouses or among the humble dwellings of those with mental health problems. Her study revealed a nineteenth-century blueprint for mental health care and treatment based on good food, exercise, fresh air, meaningful occupation, entertainment and diversionary activities as well as spiritual care in an aesthetically pleasing environment. This blueprint had originated from the work of the Quaker William Tuke, who established the York Retreat at the end of the seventeenth century. Asylums were built to strict criteria based on ideas of architecture to promote sanity. Male attendants and female nurses were chosen for their ability to work alongside patients and to contribute to their quality of life. They were also to model rational thought and acceptable behaviour conforming to the social mores of the time. Additionally, there were very few therapeutic drugs of any note, most for that period being prescribed for physical illnesses. Control and order were maintained by the blueprint outlined above with very little recourse to restraint or seclusion. If the records can be believed, incidences of restraint and seclusion were fewer than in contemporary practice pro rata. Indeed the Lunacy Commission, established by the Lunatics Act 1845, oversaw the standards of care and treatment and the activities of Asylum Visitors (local magistrates). Magistrates on asylum committees visited their local asylums fortnightly, and in the early years following the compulsory establishment of county asylums, before their populations swelled exponentially, would speak with each patient to ascertain their evaluation of their treatment.

Smith and Aslan (Chapter 9 of this book) have located most of their criticisms of the history of mental health care in the period before 'moral treatment'. Carpenter does not deny that abuses existed, but argued that these were considerably fewer than we have been led to believe. She also suggested that the period which followed her study became increasingly subject to the influence of the medical model and was experimental – with nurses' roles adjusting accordingly, not necessarily for the better. While Foucault and Scull decried the entire asylum era, finding it wanting, Goffman, although generalizing beyond his research, at least referred to the contemporary situation he observed. His view is supported by oral histories such as Derek McCarthy's *Certified and Detained*, published in 2009, about his experiences as a student psychiatric nurse in the 1960s.

Notwithstanding the criticisms of the asylum era and the extent to which they were accurate, the care of the mentally ill changed according to the prevailing dominant ideologies of the day. The belief in the 'magic bullet' of chlorpromazine resulted in an increased admission rate and a change to mental health legislation. Why keep people out of psychiatric hospitals when they could be treated successfully and returned to the community? The power of psychiatry was arguably at its peak during this period and the Mental Health Act 1959 gave increased power to psychiatrists to detain people, where earlier magistrates were the principal decision-makers in this respect. Unfortunately the available treatment approaches failed to return as many people to the community as had been hoped for and populations of inpatients swelled. Coinciding with Goffman's appraisal of the total institution and the rise in the anti-psychiatry movement, eventually, along with a further change in legislation (Mental Health Act 1983) and economic crisis, the political ideology returned to the position espoused by Enoch Powell over 20 years earlier. Community care was back on the agenda. Anti-psychiatry and the post-modern and Marxist theorists challenging the status quo led to a renewed interest in the therapeutic milieu and humanism. Echoes of the asylum era before the First World War perhaps?

Psychiatric nurses became mental health nurses, arguably reflecting the move from the dominant medical model approach to embrace the more eclectic care that was being provided. In Chapter 77 of *The Craft of Caring* Poppy Buchanan Barker (2009) described the last 20 years of the twentieth century as demonstrating a shift towards working 'with people'. It could be argued that this approach had been reclaimed. The period 1845–1914 saw attendants and nurses working with the mentally ill – alongside them in so many aspects of their everyday lives. Had the medical model been responsible for the shift away from working 'with' patients to working as doctors' handmaidens? And did the changes between the 1960s and 1980s set the scene for nurses wanting to become more independent and to be considered as more professional? This chapter cannot cover the complete history of our profession, but the issues raised so far can be applied more broadly. The optional activities in this chapter will help you to achieve this.

Reflective Exercise 10.1

You may wish to read the history of your profession or some aspect of it. Nolan (1993) is a good place to start, or, if you are more interested in policy and legislation, Kathleen Jones' (1993) *Asylums and After*. Several asylums, mental or psychiatric hospitals have their own histories published: Catharine Arnold's (2008) or Paul Chamber's (2009) studies of Bedlam, Steven Cherry's (2003) account of a Norwich asylum and John Crammer's (1990) research of Buckinghamshire's County Lunatic Asylum are examples. Alternatively you may find oral testimonies such as Derek McCarthy's (2009) or Stephen Burrow's (2010) more to your taste. There are also several relevant journal articles, for example Neil Brimblecombe's published research (2005, 2006). When you have decided on your reading material, select a chapter or two, or a journal article, read it and ask yourself the following questions:

- How is the past represented?
- Is the author's representation fair? Does the author draw on primary research (their own study) or on secondary sources (others' research)?
- Is the research put into historical context? Does the author, for example, compare his or her findings with what was normal for society at the time? An example might be the diet provided in a nineteenth-century asylum. This may appear limited to our contemporary standards but when compared with paupers' diets at home or in the workhouse it was far superior in most cases.
- Does the author make generalizations based on limited examples? What occurred in one hospital might not be the same in every other hospital, so you should be cautious if the author suggests this as a truism.

Alternatively, consider these questions in relation to the extract from Carpenter's thesis in Box 10.1.

Box 10.1

Extract from Carpenter (2010, pp. 170–3)

The maintenance of order within the asylum was of paramount importance to the Visitors and the Commissioners in Lunacy (C.I.L.), a state of reasonable quietude being an indication of a well-ordered institution. William Ellis (1838, pp. 193–4) described the deliberate control of patients by withholding exercise for those for whom quietude was a desired state, and by manipulating behaviour by a system of giving or withholding rewards for those who were too quiet. John Kirkman (1794–1887), Medical Superintendent of the Suffolk County Lunatic Asylum at Woodbridge between 1831 and 1876, believed that 'Extreme quietude ... is but an uncertain criterion of the state of an Asylum, and it is difficult to understand why it should now be a test in such high estimation'. He held that an elevated or subdued tone of voice neither advanced nor diminished the patient's real comfort and illustrated his point by reference to a patient of his whose morning exercise 'is to run into the middle of the airing ground, and scream as loudly as she can ...'. He suggested that (italics original) *'it is not the persons of such patients*, but our own anticipations of quietness that must be laid under restraint ...' and that alterations [in states of quietude] were not necessarily improvements in their management (Hunter and Macalpine 1963, p. 884). Ellis and Kirkman, then, were at odds in their consideration of the importance of quietude as a desirable state and it would appear that the latter was at odds with most other contemporary influential figures, as indeed he implied. This is supported by the frequency of reporting on the

continued ➢

degree of noisiness in the local asylums of Hampshire and Portsmouth. On Boxing Day 1853 Lord Henry Cholmondeley, Chairman of the Hampshire County Lunatic Asylum (HCLA) Visitors, reported that 'the Wards were clean and orderly, & the Patients quiet' (Visitor's Report 1853). In Portsmouth in 1881, the C.I.L. reported that 'The behaviour of the patients was not altogether satisfactory, there was a good deal of noise and excitement in one or two of the wards in each division, partly due, no doubt, to the unfavourable state of the weather for outdoor exercise'. Similarly, the following year, the Commissioners reported of the Borough of Portsmouth Lunatic Asylum (BPLA) that 'Generally the patients were quiet and orderly, but the exception was in the female acute ward where some of the women became noisy and violent' (C.I.L. Annual Reports 1881, 1882).

How, then, given the prevailing opinion against the use of mechanical restraint, was the desired state of quietude achieved? Scull (1979, p. 118) supported the view of Ellis (above) when he suggested that, as medical superintendents became better accustomed to managing increased asylum populations, they began to realize that they could do without mechanical restraint by the manipulation of small rewards and privileges, seclusion, or the threat of removal to a 'worse' ward, and consequently more overtly punitive strategies were seldom required. Nolan (1993, pp. 42–4), however, identified the practical problems facing those who wanted to abolish physical means of restraint. His perspective was that severe asylum overcrowding meant that, even where restraint was not used, seclusion and solitary confinement were necessary to control refractory patients. He added that many public asylum superintendents and private madhouse proprietors used padded cells for violent patients. Scull's terminology appears to illuminate the contemporary attitude that seclusion was a positive alternative to restraint, although he continued to offer his personal view that this aspect of 'moral treatment' disguised 'a monotonous reality in which the needs of the patients were necessarily subordinated to those of the institution' (Scull 1979, p. 118). Nolan's perspective supports the view that seclusion was an equally disagreeable alternative to restraint and to reinforce Scull's personal perspective. He also appeared to use the terms 'seclusion' and 'solitary confinement' interchangeably, while Conolly (1856) was clear about the differences in practice:

> [seclusion] is not to be ascribed to want of opportunities of observation that such a simple exclusion of irritations from an irritable mind, an exclusion not found to be necessary in more than four or five instances in any one day in the year among a thousand patients, and seldom prolonged beyond four or five hours in any of those instances, during which time the patient's state is frequently ascertained by means of the inspection-plate on the door of his room, and all his reasonable wants and wishes are attended to, should ever have been confounded with the idea of solitary confinement – the latter in reality comprehending a privation of almost all the stimuli upon which the integrity of intellectual and physical life depends.

The HCLA Visitors in 1853 remarked that 'the patients are generally tranquil and no one was under mechanical restraint. Such restraint indeed has never been employed nor has seclusion of the patients been resorted to except in rare instances'. Just a month later, however, the report was rather different: 'We have this day visited the Asylum and have seen all the patients – None were [sic] under restraint, but several were in seclusion' (HCLA, Visitor's Report 1853). A year later, Dr Manley recorded that:

> *The seclusion of Patients, for a short period, is resorted to for two purposes:- first, as a calmative to allay excitability, by the removal of all sources of extraneous irritation, for which purpose it is a valuable remedial means; and, secondly, to isolate, during excitement, a patient who is occasionally an annoyance to several, if not all, the others in the same ward. The seclusions during the last six months on the Male side have been very inconsiderable, and on the Female side are each of short duration, and confined to a few Patients.*
>
> (Medical Superintendent's Annual Report 1854, p. 16)

Reporting the incidents of seclusion at the HCLA in 1871, he sought to justify its continuance:

> *There are a few Patients here of so dangerous a character that it is sometimes necessary to resort to seclusion to prevent accidents. Not long ago, a man who had been sent here as a Criminal Lunatic attempted, taking advantage of the position of an Attendant, to gouge out one of his eyes. He had previously attacked three other persons in succession, cutting another Attendant in the face; and there have been several other Patients under treatment during the past 12 months with strong homicidal propensities.*
>
> (Medical Superintendent's Annual Report 1871, p. 17)

The phrase 'resort to seclusion' suggests that it was not seen locally as a positive or desirable alternative to restraint, as Scull suggested was the common view, but a necessary evil, a view consistent with Nolan's interpretation of events.

Reflective Exercise 10.2

Select a period in recent history and consider mental health policy, legislation and practice in the context of political, economic and social changes. You may wish further to consider another period of history and repeat the exercise. Can you see a pattern?

Alternatively, consider these aspects as you read the extract from the 1885 edition of the *Handbook For The Instruction Of Attendants on the Insane* about 'precautions against suicide' in Box 10.2

Box 10.2

Extract from *Handbook For The Instruction Of Attendants on the Insane* (Campbell *et al.* 1885, p. 51)

When the suicidal propensity is known or suspected, the Doctor usually gives instructions for the Patient to be placed under special observation – that is, to be kept under the

continued ➤

direct and constant observation of one or other of the Attendants. When this order is given, the Attendant should carry it out faithfully. There should be no negligence, no allowing the Patient to wander away from the room and get out of sight for a longer or shorter time, and no relaxing of watchfulness without direct permission from the Doctor, for there is no knowing when or how a suicidal Patient will attempt to carry out his intention. In passing him from the charge of one to another, the first Attendant should, before relinquishing duty, see that the second Attendant has duly taken him under his care. Such articles as scissors, razors, knives etc., which may be used for suicidal purposes, should be carefully kept out of the Patient's way. It is well to have these articles safely locked up when not in use. They should be counted when given out for use, and again when taken back, so as to ensure that none are [sic] left out. All medicines should be kept in a place of safety. It may be necessary to examine the Patient's pockets and clothing at frequent times, to see that he has not succeeded in secreting anything that may be used hurtfully.

Barker (2009, p. 732) debated professional values and referred to Florence Nightingale's fundamental philosophical principle of avoiding iatrogenesis, that is, the hospital (including the nurse) should do the sick no harm (Nightingale 1863). Yet Barker also outlined chilling examples of nurses' involvement in the atrocities of the holocaust and how, when they were called to account, they declared that they were just following orders. Nurses, Barker illustrated, gave other rationalizations for causing harm to others including their 'beliefs' that they were bringing a welcome end to miserable lives. Harold Shipman believed similarly when he killed (or hastened the deaths of) many of his patients. Debates continue to rage about nurses' involvement in assisted suicide and on the extent to which they may conscientiously object to participating in practices they find abhorrent or which contradict their values, beliefs and integrity.

The 'what now?' of mental health nursing

In turning our attention to the 'what now' of mental health nursing, the NMC code (2008) includes the requirement that as a nurse you must:

- Make the care of people your first concern, treating them as individuals and respecting their dignity
- Work with others to protect and promote the health and wellbeing of those in your care, their families and carers, and the wider community
- Provide a high standard of practice and care at all times
- Be open and honest, act with integrity and uphold the reputation of your profession.

The code (NMC 2008) also states that, as professionals, nurses are personally accountable for actions and omissions in their practice and must always be able to justify their decisions and act lawfully, whether those laws relate to their professional practice or personal life.

Similarly, the NMC (2010) standards for pre-registration nursing education arguably provide the current blueprint for *baseline* standards and competencies for mental health nursing. Mental health nurses must, for instance, work with people of all ages using values-based mental health frameworks. Indeed, nursing curricula are being based on these very principles (see Chapter 3). But what does it really mean? How straightforward is it to use values-based mental health frameworks? The NMC (2010) qualified its statement thus:

> *They must use different methods of engaging people, and work in a way that promotes positive relationships focused on social inclusion, human rights and recovery, that is, a person's ability to live a self-directed life, with or without symptoms, that they believe is meaningful and satisfying.*
>
> *(p. 22)*

Presumably the 'they' the NMC refers to are service users and not mental health nurses. What happens though if a service user's standard of a meaningful and satisfying life is different from ours, or if theirs or ours differs from that of the government? The Department of Health's (DH's) latest strategy for mental health *No Health Without Mental Health* (2011) outlines its principles for high-quality care. It includes: 'putting the person at the centre and sharing decision making – "No decision about me without me" should be a governing principle in service design and delivery' (p. 32). This is certainly laudable on paper, but consider the extent to which it is consistent with the DH blueprint for mental health based on the Foresight Report (Government Office for Science 2008), which recommends five ways to mental wellbeing:

1. **Connect** with the people around you, family, friends, colleagues and neighbours
2. **Be active** – go for a walk or a run, garden, play a game
3. **Take notice** – be curious and aware of the world around you
4. **Keep learning** – try a new recipe, learn a new language, set yourself a challenge
5. **Give** – do something nice for somebody, volunteer, join a community group.

Chapter 3 has exercises on the topic of values-based practice. This present chapter, however, is more concerned with the critical analysis of the concepts and practice of mental health nursing past and present and, in turn, lessons that may be taken into the future. With this difference in mind consider the following reflective exercise.

Reflective Exercise 10.3

Think about a person with mental health problems that you know or whom you have nursed:

- To what extent were they able to achieve the five ways to mental wellbeing identified in bold above?

continued ➤

- If they were not able to attain any of these areas, what were the barriers and how could (or did) nursing intervention help?
- Do you think the person you are remembering shared these values?
- Are you able to achieve these ideals in your own life and do you agree with them?
- Can you think of any you would like to add?
- How different is this blueprint from that which underpinned nineteenth-century practice identified above, namely good food, exercise, fresh air, meaningful occupation, entertainment and diversionary activities, as well as spiritual care, in an aesthetically pleasing environment?

The NMC (2010) maintains that:

Mental health nurses must practise in such a way that promotes self-determination and expertise of people with mental health problems, using a range of approaches and tools that aid wellness and recovery and enable self-care and self-management.

(p. 28)

Indeed throughout the NMC document the standards and competencies for mental health nurses refer to promoting service user determination, wellness, recovery and evidence-based practice. This chapter began with reference to a question by Barker about whether the emergent concept of 'recovery' was the final destination of care or the latest fashion. Similar questions may be raised of evidence-based and values-based practice (see Chapters 6 and 3, respectively). Are these also fashions, however, soon to be replaced by newer fads? On one hand it could be argued that evidence-based practice has been superseded by values-based practice. On the other hand perhaps evidence-based practice has become so integral to nursing care that we do not talk or write about it so often. In the 1970s the Nursing Process was the newest fashion, but now, other than teaching it to new students, it barely receives notice. It is as difficult to imagine not assessing patients, planning and implementing their care and evaluating the outcomes as it is to contemplate providing a non-evidence-based intervention. Before evidence-based practice became commonplace, rarely did local or even national policies base their recommendations or standards on research or other forms of evidence. In contemporary health care, the National Institute for Health and Clinical Excellence (NICE) guidelines, for example, provide a key to the types of evidence on which their recommendations are made so that practitioners, in turn, may be confident in educating and informing people about them and encouraging health behaviour and engagement with interventions and services consistent with them.

Reflective Exercise 10.4

This is a library-based exercise which requires you to do a bit of detective work. Seek out a policy from the 1970s or 1980s and look for reference to research-based or other forms of evidence which guided its recommendations. Compare this with one of the current NICE guidelines or a contemporary policy.

- Do you think evidence-based practice has become more integrated into contemporary health care?
- Are the sources of evidence more transparent today than 30 or 40 years ago?

Returning to the question of whether values-based practice has supplanted evidence-based practice, might it not be, therefore, that we need to make less frequent reference to the latter as it has become embedded within contemporary mental health nursing practice? This raises further questions, however. First, has nursing practice become unbalanced in favour of scientific evidence to the exclusion of 'values' and other markers of humanism? Second, is values-based practice really new or had we forgotten it – only to rediscover it anew now? In either case it would suggest that underpinning philosophies may become so integral to our practice that we forget to explain them and pass them on to our successors, therefore over time they become lost and must be revived. How similar is the values-based practice approach outlined in Chapter 3 to the humanistic principles of Carl Rogers (1951) of the belief in the uniqueness and worth of each individual, non-judgemental attitudes, non-possessive warmth, unconditional positive regard and empathy, which formed the basis of psychiatric nursing curricula and practice in the 1970s and 1980s (see also Chapter 2)? Is it not likely that contemporary and indeed future mental health nursing should be a healthy mix of both evidence-based and values-based approaches?

Similar discussions may be had about wellness and recovery. Are the expectations that service users are central to their recovery process and continued wellness any different from the attitudes and beliefs that prompted and promoted community care 30 or more years ago? Earlier in this chapter the effect of poor historical practice on our image of the past was raised. In that scenario one of the main failings was the lack of contextualization of past practices – of viewing them with our contemporary knowledge, skills and attitudes rather than in their true historical past. Thus to understand past practice we must consider the political, economic and social climate of the day. It is no different with contemporary practice. We must, for example, therefore consider recovery and community-based care (in all its forms) in the light of the political, economic and social climate.

Think about the political, economic and social changes in our recent history and today. What was the prevailing political agenda and how did it inform mental health policy. Compare, perhaps, the *National Service Framework for Mental Health* (NSF; DH 1999), *New Horizons* (DH 2009) and *No Health Without Mental Health* (DH 2011). The NSF and *New Horizons* were both Labour government initiatives.

- How similar were they?
- How can any differences be accounted for?
- What was happening economically and socially at the time each was published?
- How different from them is the Coalition government's latest policy *No Health Without Mental Health* and why?

Given your engagement with Reflexive Exercise 10.5, you might now contemplate the extent to which each of these approaches, philosophies or types of mental health practice are fads of fashion or understandable entities in the broader context in which they arose. Is this any different from fashion? Is it always progressive? This last question is particularly interesting when you consider the number of initiatives that appear to re-emerge over time, newly packaged and labelled. Are they principally the same or similar products but with added, new and improved features? Recovery is not a new idea. Following the lunacy laws of 1845, statistics were submitted to the government annually of those discharged from county asylums 'recovered', 'relieved' or 'not improved'. It can be argued that recovery has always been an ideal. There is never enough money in the Exchequer to detain people, delay their recovery or treat them unnecessarily, at least within the National Health Service (NHS). So commonplace words such as 'recovery' take on different meanings in their variable contexts. Contemporary 'recovery' is then, perhaps, a newly packaged and improved take on a relatively consistent concept. The context is all important. Not least in keeping abreast of changes and advocating for developments in the face of counter-arguments and negative attitudes by those who have 'seen it all before'.

This need for contextualization may also help to make sense of the challenges to mental health nursing. In 2009, Barker discussed the (fight) between mental health nurses and the new breed of mental health practitioner to claim 'caring' and 'therapeutic being' as their own (pp. 734–5). He raised concerns that mental health nursing would be lost or sidelined. The Mental Health Practitioner (MHP) programme to which he referred was developed in response to a shortage in mental health nurses and local recruitment problems. Before long the situations became filled, the skill-mix became saturated with MHPs and the local Trusts ceased to commission their training. This was not the whole picture as the political climate was changing and the economy was facing another crisis.

MHPs themselves had difficulty in defining the way in which their practice was unique from other professional groups within mental health care, a stumbling block to them being able to achieve professional status in their own right. The fight to become professionally regulated has most recently been achieved by psychologists, before that by occupational therapists. In the 1970s psychiatric nurses complained that occupational therapists working within mental health care had usurped an important part of their role. Indeed providing meaningful occupation had been absolutely integral and exclusive to nursing the mentally ill from the mid-nineteenth to mid-twentieth centuries. Have not mental health nurses, however, equally been responsible for treading on the toes of other mental health professionals? For example, nurses are increasingly developing further skills in cognitive behavioural therapy (CBT) and dialectical behavioural therapy (DBT), the sometime province of psychologists. Other extended roles give nurses the opportunity to prescribe medication (within limits) overlapping with the essence of medical practice. The 2007 amendments to the Mental Health Act allow nurses (and other registered mental health professionals), after further training, to assume the role of Approved Mental Health Professional, one-time exclusive to Approved Social Workers.

The 'what next?' of mental health nursing

History is the study of change over time. Some changes are radical, usually at times of war or economic crises, whereas others are more incremental. It is perhaps unsurprising then that the role of the mental health nurse should have changed over time, having lost some aspects and gained others. But what will become of it in the future? *No Health Without Mental Health* outlines six underpinning objectives to its strategy for contemporary mental health care (DH 2011):

1. More people will have good mental health
2. More people with mental health problems will recover
3. More people with mental health problems will have good physical health
4. More people will have a positive experience of care and support
5. Fewer people will suffer avoidable harm
6. Fewer people will experience stigma and discrimination.

Perhaps two significant areas impacting on the future of mental health nursing, related to the above objectives and integral to the policy, are, first, the developing role of Increasing Access to Psychological Therapies (IAPT) services and, second, the prevention of illhealth. IAPT is currently a primarycare-based service built on principles of CBT for people with mild to moderate anxiety and depression to more extreme forms of mental health difficulty. Stepped care is provided from low-intensity to high-intensity intervention through a variety of media from face-to-face to telephone interaction or computer-based self-help modalities. Its success over time (and its specific and individualistic evidence base) is yet to be evaluated. Notwithstanding this, the Coalition government (and the Labour government which preceded it) has welcomed it and is interested in its role beyond primary care and for more people with a greater variety of mental health problems. Is this another fad or can it be seen in the context of expedience in economically straitened times? Certainly the low-intensity interventions are usually offered over five or six sessions of up to half an hour's duration. If this proves to be as or more successful than medication or other forms of treatment and is acceptable to service users, then who can argue with it?

Reflective Exercise 10.6

- What do you think could be the potential impact of IAPT services on contemporary mental health nursing?
- Is this an area that mental health nurses could develop and add to their repertoire?
- Is it a service that encourages reflexive practice?
- Alternatively, should mental health nurses focus more upon the care of those traditionally difficult to engage with 'talking' therapies, those who have, to coin a well-used phrase, more serious and disabling mental health problems?

The second area of note from the latest mental health strategy is the prevention of illhealth. Indeed this is the fourth domain of the first objective. The third objective, as identified above, is that more people with mental health problems will have good physical health (DH 2011). The policy focuses on reducing the numbers of people with mental health problems who develop preventable physical problems. This refers to those conditions which are lifestyle related (whether or not as a consequence of mental health problems) as well as those which could have been prevented by better observation, care and screening. Mental health nurses certainly have a role and responsibility in this regard. Research reported in May 2011 stated that people with serious mental illnesses such as schizophrenia, bipolar disorder or those being treated for substance misuse can have a life expectancy 10–15 years lower than the UK average. The research was carried out by the Biomedical Research Centre for Mental Health at Maudsley Hospital in London. The researchers believed a combination of factors – higherrisk lifestyles, long-term anti-psychotic drug use and social disadvantage – could be to blame (Hughes 2011).

> **Reflective Exercise 10.7**
>
> Think of a service user with whom you have recently worked who has complex needs.
>
> - Does this person have any physical health problems at the moment?
> - In what way might their lifestyle contribute to risk for future physical health problems?
> - To what extent are these factors preventable?
> - Can you identify potential barriers to preventing physical illhealth?
> - How might you work with the service user to overcome these?

When seeking to identify ourselves as mental health nurses, we often define ourselves with respect to the erosion of our role, rather than, as discussed above, any extensions to it that we have gained. Similarly, perhaps we forget the tradition of nursing to which we belong. While others may work therapeutically with service users, how holistically is this achieved? Are other practitioners trained to recognize the physical health problems that so frequently co-exist with mental health problems? In this respect, how at risk are we of losing, ignoring or failing to develop these skills ourselves? The NMC standards for pre-registration nursing (2010) retained distinct fields of nursing, but only just. The curricula currently being written to those standards seek to integrate the fields where possible, as well as taking advantage of other inter-professional learning with related disciplines. Some curricula are offering dual fields in adult and mental health nursing. It is likely that graduates from such a course will be very well placed to promote health improvement and reduce preventable mortality for those with mental health problems. Such an integrated approach to caring for people with mental and physical health problems is not unique. Indeed globally it is more common to combine the two, albeit with different levels of success as the World Health Organization frequently testifies. However, if mental health nurses adapt to the contexts in which they find themselves, and the current context finds service users dying between 10 and 15 years earlier than necessary, then, arguably, this is the current context we must embrace and address.

The NMC (2010) maintained that:

All nurses must be self-aware and recognise how their own values, principles and assumptions may affect their practice. They must maintain their own personal and professional development, learning from experience, through supervision, feedback, reflection and evaluation.

(p. 29)

If mental health nurses are going to achieve their ongoing professional development they must move with the times. They must analyse their own practice and check for contextual consistency with current best practice, ensuring both evidence-based and values-based approaches.

> **Reflective Exercise 10.8**
>
> Consider the NMC statement above, and your reading of preceding chapters in this book, and reflect upon your values, principles and assumptions and how these might affect your practice. How might you ensure that you remain professionally uptodate and that your practice is consistent with the contemporary context in which you find yourself?

Conclusion

This chapter, then, has considered the 'what then, what now, what next' of mental health nursing. This examination has seen the reinvention of a wheel or two, but arguably with refinements and improvements. It has encouraged a questioning approach to the representation of our past as strongly as we would wish to question current practice. Some of the challenges to the role of the mental health nurse have been considered and to a cautious extent the direction of travel it faces in the future has been predicted. What remains fairly certain is that ongoing change is inevitable and that we must move with it and, moreover, seek to influence it.

References

Arnold C (2008) *Bedlam: London and Its Mad*. London: Simon and Schuster.

Barker P (ed.) (2009) *Psychiatric and Mental Health Nursing: The Craft of Caring*, 2nd edn. London: Hodder Arnold.

Brimblecombe N (2005) Asylum nursing in the UK at the end of the Victorian era: Hill End Asylum. *Journal of Psychiatric and Mental Health Nursing* **12**, 57–63.

Brimblecombe N (2006) Asylum nursing as a career in the United Kingdom, 1890–1910. *Journal of Advanced Nursing* **55**, 770–7.

Buchanan Barker P (2009) Reclamation: beyond recovery, in Barker P (ed.) *Psychiatric and Mental Health Nursing: The Craft of Caring*, 2nd edn. London: Hodder Arnold.

Burrows S (2010) *Buddleia Dance on the Asylum: A Nurse's Journey Through a Mental Hospital*. Cambridge: Melrose Books.

Campbell Clark A, McIvor Campbell C, Turnbull AR, Urquhart AR (1885) *Handbook for the Instruction of Attendants on the Insane (1885)*. London: Bailliere Tindall and Cox.

Carpenter D (2010) *Above All a Patient Should Never be Terrified: An Examination of Mental Health Care and Treatment in Hampshire*, 1845–1914. Unpublished PhD thesis, University of Portsmouth.

Carroll L (1907) *Alice's Adventures in Wonderland*. London: William Heinemann.

Chambers P (2009) *Bedlam: London's Hospital for the Mad*. Weybridge: Ian Allan Publishing.

Cherry S (2003) *Mental Health Care in Modern England: The Norfolk Lunatic Asylum/ St Andrew's Hospital c.1810–1998.* Woodbridge: Boydell Press.

Conolly J (1856) *Treatment of the Insane without Mechanical Restraints.* London: Dawsons of Pall Mall (reprinted 1973).

Crammer J (1990) *Asylum History: Buckinghamshire County Pauper Lunatic Asylum – St John's.* London: Gaskell.

DH (1999) *National Service Framework for Mental Health: Modern Standards and Service Models.* London: The Stationery Office.

DH (2009) *New Horizons.* London: The Stationery Office.

DH (2011) *No Health Without Mental Health.* London: The Stationery Office.

Driscoll J (1994) Reflective practice for practise – a framework of structured reflection for clinical areas. *Senior Nurse* **14**(1), 47–50.

Ellis WC (1838) *A Treatise on the Nature, Symptoms, Causes, and Treatment of Insanity, with Practical Observation on Lunatic Asylums, and a Description of the Pauper Lunatic Asylum for the County of Middlesex at Hanwell, with a Detailed Account of its Management.* London: Holdsworth.

Foucault M (2001) *Madness and Civilization: A History of Insanity in the Age of Reason*, trans. R Howard. London: Routledge (first published in 1967 by Tavistock Publications).

Foucault M (2006) *Psychiatric Power: Lectures at the College De France, 1973–74*, English series ed. AI Davidson, trans. G Burchell. Basingstoke: Palgrave Macmillan.

Gardner L, Rolfe G (2009) The possibility of genuine mental health nursing, in Barker P (ed.) *Psychiatric and Mental Health Nursing: The Craft of Caring*, 2nd edn. London: Hodder Arnold.

Goffman E (1961) *Asylums: Essays on the Social Situation of Mental Patients and Other Inmates.* London: Penguin Books.

Government Office for Science (2008) *Mental Capital and Wellbeing: Making the Most of Ourselves in the 21st Century – Final Project Report.* Online: http://tinyurl.com/ ForesightReportMentalCapital (accessed 20 June 2011).

Hughes D (2011) *Mentally Ill Have Reduced Life Expectancy, Study Finds.* Online http://www. bbc.co.uk/news/health-13414965 (accessed:18 May 2011).

Hunter R, Macalpine I (1963) *Three Hundred Years of Psychiatry 1535–1860.* Oxford: Oxford University Press.

Jones K (1993) *Asylums and After.* London: Continuum.

Lunatics Act (1845) 8 and 9 Vict. c. 100. An Act for the Regulation of the Care and Treatment of Lunatics 1845.

McCarthy D (2009) *Certified and Detained: The True Story of Life in a UK Mental Hospital from 1957 to 1963 as Seen Then Through the Eyes of a Male Student Nurse.* Privately published by D & L McCarthy Products (available through Amazon Books, www. amazon.co.uk/books).

Mental Health Act (1959) Elizabeth II, Chapter 42. London: The Stationery Office.

Mental Health Act (1983) Elizabeth II, Chapter 20. London: The Stationery Office.

Mental Health Act (2007) Elizabeth II, Chapter 12. London: The Stationery Office.

Nightingale F (1863) *Notes on Hospitals,* 3rd edn. London: Longman.

NMC (2008) *The Code: Standards of Conduct, Performance and Ethics for Nurses and Midwives*. London: Nursing and Midwifery Council. Online: www.nmc-uk.org/Nurses-and-midwives/The-code/The-code-in-full/ (accessed 24 June 2011).

NMC (2010) *Standards for Pre-Registration Nursing Education*. London: Nursing and Midwifery Council.

Nolan P (1993) *A History of Mental Health Nursing*. London: Chapman and Hall.

Rogers C (1951) *Client-centred Therapy*. Boston, MA: Houghton-Mifflin.

Santayana G (1920) *The Life of Reason, Or The Phases of Human Progress Volume 1*. New York, NY: Charles Scribner's Sons.

Scull A (1979) *Museums of Madness: The Social Organization of Insanity in Nineteenth Century England*. London: Allen Lane.

Sick Britain: Urban Exploration (2009) *Top 10 Abandoned Asylums*. Online: www.sickbritain.co.uk/2009/08/top-10-abandoned-asylums-in-the-uk (accessed 20 May 2011).

Tosh J (2008) *Why History Matters*. Basingstoke: Palgrave Macmillan.

Primary documentary sources

Hampshire Record Office (1853) 48M94/A1/1, HCLA, *Committee of Visitors Minute Book, Visitors Report*, 26 December.

Hampshire Record Office (1854) 48M94/A9/1, HCLA, *Annual Report of the Medical Superintendent* (A.R.M.S.), p. 16

Hampshire Record Office (1871) 48M94/A9/2, HCLA, A.R.M.S., p. 17.

Portsmouth City Records Office (1881, 1882) PR/H8/1/7/1, BPLA, *Commissioners in Lunacy Annual Reports*.

Index